Foot and Ankle Disorders
Tricks of the Trade

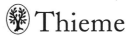

Foot and Ankle Disorders
Tricks of the Trade

Frederick G. Lippert III, M.D.

Professor of Surgery and Head Division of Orthopaedic Surgery
Department of Surgery
Uniformed Services University of The Health Sciences
Residency Program Director
Department of Orthopaedics
National Naval Medical Center
Bethesda, MD

Sigvard T. Hansen Jr., M.D.

Professor and Chairman Emeritus
Department of Orthopaedics
University of Washington
Seattle, WA

Thieme
New York • Stuttgart

BS

Acquisitions Editor: Esther Gumpert
Director, Production and Manufacturing: Anne Vinnicombe
Production Editor: Anne Vinnicombe
Marketing Director: Phyllis Gold
Sales Director: Ross Lumpkin
Chief Financial Officer: Peter van Woerden
President: Brian Scanlan
Compositor: Sallyann Hobson
Printer: Sheridan Books

Library of Congress Cataloging-in-Publication Data is available from the publisher.

Important note: Medical knowledge is ever-changing. As new research and clinical experience broaden our knowledge, changes in treatment and drug therapy may be required. The author of the material herein has consulted sources believed to be reliable in her efforts to provide information that is complete and in accord with standards accepted at the time of publication. However, in view of the possibility of human error by the author or publisher of the work herein, or changes in medical knowledge, neither the author nor the publisher, nor any other party who has been involved in the preparation of this work, warrants that the information contained herein is in every respect accurate or complete, and they are not responsible for any errors or omissions or for the results obtained by the use of such information. Readers are advised to check the product information sheet included in the package of each drug they plan to administer to be certain that the information contained in this publication is accurate and that changes have not been made in the recommended dose or in the contraindications for administration. This recommendation is of particular importance in connection with new and infrequently used drugs.

Some of the product names, patents, and registered designs referred to in this book are in fact registered trademarks or proprietary names even though specific reference to this fact

is not always made in the text. Therefore, the appearance of a name without designation as proprietary is not to be construed as a representation by the publisher that it is in the public domain.

Printed in the United States

5 4 3 2 1

TMP ISBN 1–58890–141–6

GTV ISBN 3 13 135511 5

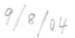
9/8/04

Contents

Preface

One day of the week-long Basic Course for Orthopaedic Educators, sponsored by the American Academy of Orthopaedic Surgeons, is devoted to teaching psychomotor skills, also known as surgical or bioskills. The participating orthopaedic surgeons are advised to keep a surgical diary as a means of recording in words and drawings their tricks of the trade for use in subsequent surgeries. These tricks and pitfalls, described in the diary after every surgery where something new is learned, provide a reference for review before they perform a given procedure the next time.

Coauthor Sigvard T. Hansen Jr. is a master surgeon who continuously improves his techniques by using tricks that he devises over time. Through my work and association with him, it occurred to me that a surgical diary built on his and my tricks of the trade could be very valuable to others. This book is just that. It is not meant to be exhaustive and all encompassing; rather it focuses on certain procedures that are associated with a steep learning curve, cause trouble, and are difficult to understand or perform.

Each chapter addresses specific procedures. The drawings are simple and straightforward. Explanatory notes, tricks, and pitfalls are next to the drawings to help the reader get the gist of each procedure at a glance.

The tricks and techniques in this book are the coauthors' and contributors' personal schema for performing various foot and ankle surgeries. We anticipate that some readers will disagree with one or another approach we recommend. Some will use this diary and build on it, and others will be motivated to write their own. We also hope this book will be helpful to others in teaching residents and educating patients, as it has been for us.

Frederick G. Lippert III

Contributors

Frederick G. Lippert III, M.D.
Professor of Surgery and Head Division of Orthopaedic Surgery
Uniformed Services University of The Health Sciences
Residency Program Director
Department of Orthopaedics
National Naval Medical Center
Bethesda, MD

Sigvard T. Hansen Jr., M.D.
Professor and Chairman Emeritus
Department of Orthopaedics
University of Washington
Seattle, WA

Richard L. Baker, D.P.M., D.A.B.P.S.
Private Practice
Cleveland, TN

Amir Fayazi, M.D.
Resident
Orthopaedic Surgery
Hershey Medical Center
Hershey, PA

Thomas Franchini, D.P.M.
Burlington, VT

Daniel Garcia Hospitalman Third Class USN
Orthopaedic Technician
National Naval Medical Center
Bethesda, MD

Edward S. Holt, M.D.
Private Practice
Annapolis, MD

Paul J. Juliano, M.D.
Associate Professor of Orthopaedic Surgery
Hershey Medical Center
Hershey, PA

Stephen Pinney, M.D., M.Ed. F.R.C.S.(C.)
Assistant Professor and Chief Orthopaedic Foot and Ankle Service
University of California–Sacramento, CA

Craig Williams, D.P.M., D.A.B.P.S.
Chief of Podiatry
National Naval Medical Center
Bethesda, MD

Acronyms

AO: Association for the Internal Fixation of Fractures
AP: anterior posterior
C-C: calcaneocuboid
CMT: Charcot-Marie-Tooth Disease
DCP: dynamic compression plate
DJD: degenerative joint disease
DMAA: distal metatarsal articular angle
EDB: extensor digitorum brevis
EDL: extensor digitorum longus
EHB: extensor hallucis brevis
EHL: extensor hallicus longus
FDB: flexor digitorum brevis
FDL: flexor digitorum longus
FHB: flexor hallicus brevis
FHL: flexor hallicus longus
IP: interphalangeal joint
MTP: metatarsal phalangeal joint
N-C: naviculocuneiform joint
PB: peroneus brevis tendon
PT: peroneus tertius tendon
PTT: posterior tibial tendon
ROM: range of motion
SPLATT: split lateral anterior tibialis transfer
TA: tibialis anterior
TMT: tarsal metatarsal joint
T-N: talonavicular joint

Chapter 1 The Foot and Ankle Surgical Support Bump

Daniel Garcia, Hospitalman Third Class USN

The "bump" is customized from four cloth and two paper towels rolled up and held by a Coband wrap. The size and shape are adjustable. This provides a soft yet stable support that holds its shape under the weight of the lower extremity; supports and holds or elevates the foot above the operating table, thereby improving visual, operative, and X-ray access for many procedures; and is easily moved and adjusted during the procedure.

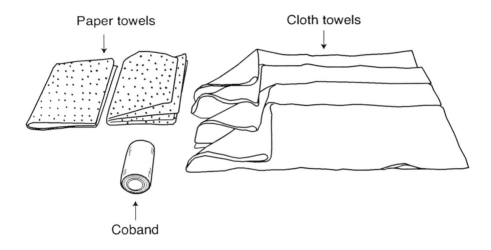

Paper towels

Cloth towels

Coband

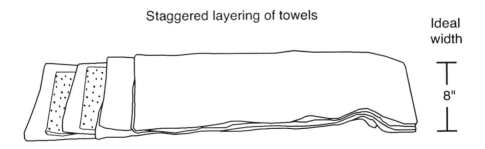

Staggered layering of towels

Ideal width

8"

Pitfalls: Bump won't support foot due to
1. Oval shape
2. Ends not being wrapped
3. Coband not wrapped tightly enough

Roll towels tightly into a cylinder

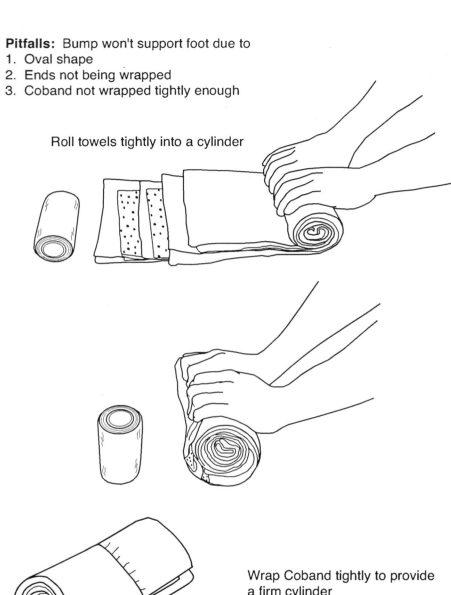

Wrap Coband tightly to provide
a firm cylinder

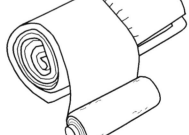

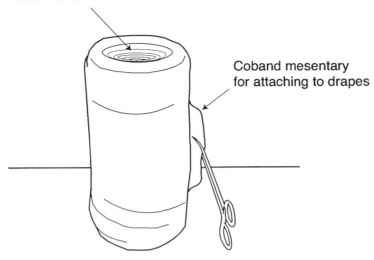

Indentation for heel

Coband mesentary for attaching to drapes

Applications of the Foot Bump

Place bump under heel or calf when applying ankle tourniquet and postoperative dressing

Coband wrap to isolate toes

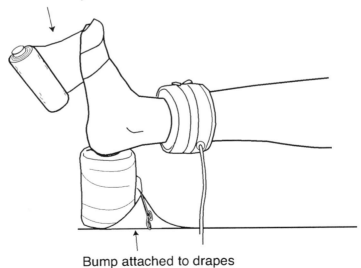

Bump attached to drapes

Chapter 1 The Foot and Ankle Surgical Support Bump   3

Place bump under knee when applying plaster splint

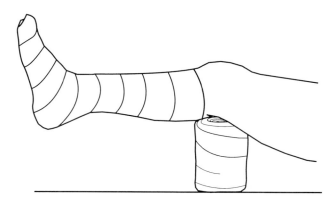

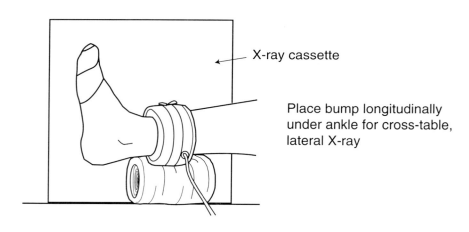

X-ray cassette

Place bump longitudinally under ankle for cross-table, lateral X-ray

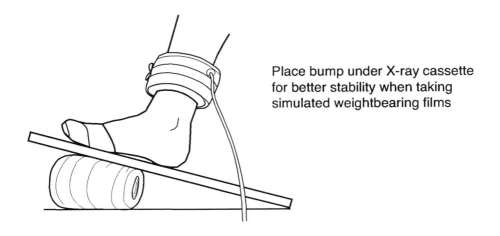

Place bump under X-ray cassette
for better stability when taking
simulated weightbearing films

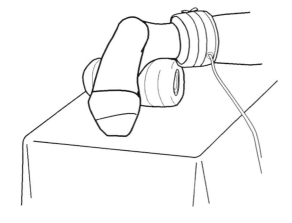

Place bump to support
foot when patient is in
prone position

Chapter 1 The Foot and Ankle Surgical Support Bump   5

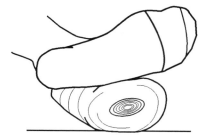

Place bump to elevate foot from operating table for better access

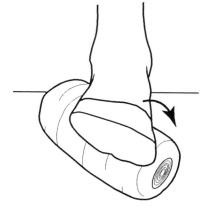

Place bump to evert foot while suturing ankle ligaments

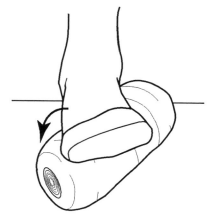

Place bump to adjust foot position during ankle ligament surgery and to invert ankle for better approach to sinus tarsi

Chapter 2 Local Anesthesia for Foot and Ankle Procedures

Frederick G. Lippert III, M.D.

Most foot and ankle anesthesia can be done with 10 to 20 mL.

Anesthetic Agents
Equal amounts:

1% Xylocaine and 0.5% Marcaine plus 1 mL of 0.84% sodium bicarbonate per 10 mL of anesthetic to avoid burning sensation

Enhancing Anesthetic Response
Tricks:
1. Inject line of incision
2. Use ankle tourniquet
3. Inject anesthetic into ligaments, capsules, and periosteum as needed during surgery

Brostrom Ankle Ligament Reconstruction

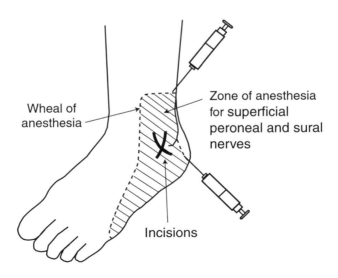

Wheal of anesthesia

Zone of anesthesia for superficial peroneal and sural nerves

Incisions

Insertional Achilles Tendinosis, Excision of Haglund's Deformity and Bony Ridges

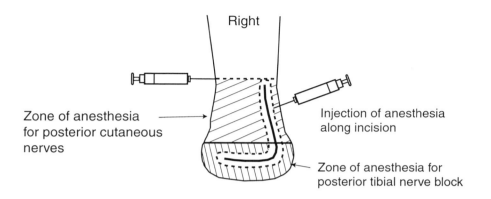

Right

Zone of anesthesia
for posterior cutaneous
nerves

Injection of anesthesia
along incision

Zone of anesthesia for
posterior tibial nerve block

Alternative to Posterior Tibial Nerve Block for Morton's Neuroma

Pitfall: Initial block unsuccessful
Trick: Web space block

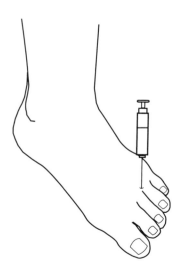

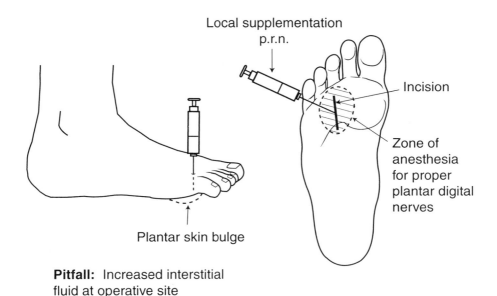

Local supplementation
p.r.n.

Incision

Zone of
anesthesia
for proper
plantar digital
nerves

Plantar skin bulge

Pitfall: Increased interstitial
fluid at operative site

Cheilectomy of Talonavicular Joint, Hardware Removal, Naviculocuneiform Fusion

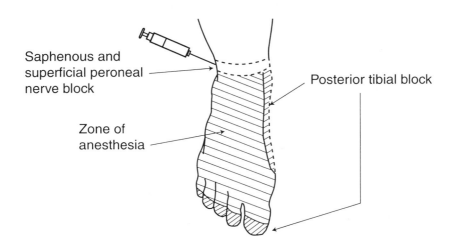

Saphenous and
superficial peroneal
nerve block

Posterior tibial block

Zone of
anesthesia

Posterior Tibial Nerve Block

Plantar Fasciotomy, Deep Hardware Removal, and Resection of Plantar Fibromatosis

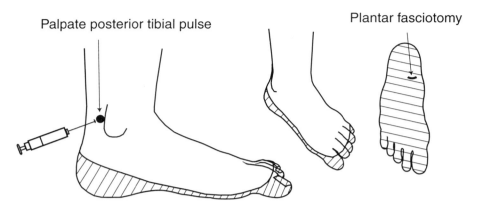

Palpate posterior tibial pulse

Plantar fasciotomy

Pitfall: Patient's foot jumps when paresthesias felt

Tricks:
1. Have assistant hold leg during injection
2. Insert needle just behind pulse and advance gently
3. Seek paresthesias
4. Inject 3 to 5 mL of anesthetic mixture at the site of paresthesias

Ankle Arthrotomy

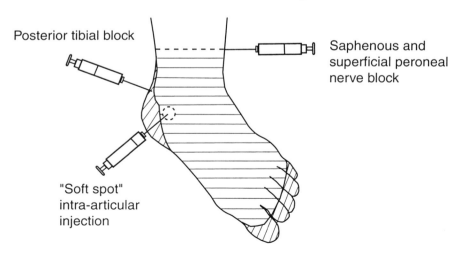

Posterior tibial block

Saphenous and superficial peroneal nerve block

"Soft spot" intra-articular injection

Naviculocuneiform and Tarsometatarsal Fusions, Debridement Posterior Tibial Tendon, Transfer of Flexor Digitorum Longus to Posterior Tibial Tendon, and Excision of the Accessory Navicular Joint

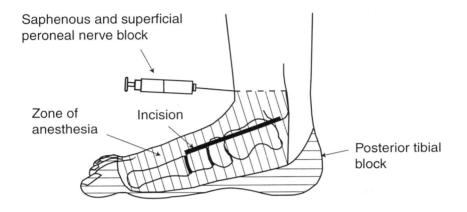

Harvest of Bone Graft from Calcaneus

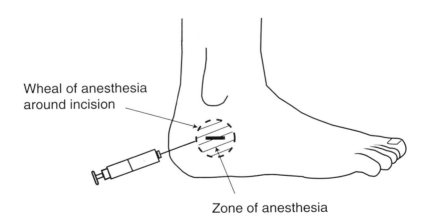

Chapter 3
Mayo Block for Hallux Procedures

Richard L. Baker, D.P.M., D.A.B.P.S.

The Mayo block is a field block around the base of the first metatarsal that involves infiltration of local anesthetic proximal to the surgical site in a ring-type fashion.

Dorsal Anatomy

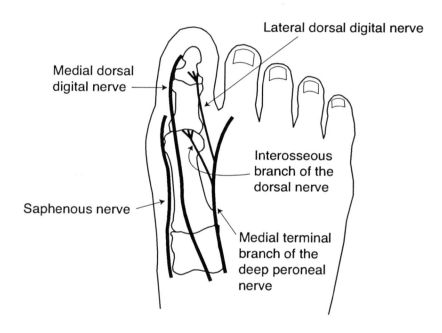

Lateral dorsal digital nerve

Medial dorsal digital nerve

Interosseous branch of the dorsal nerve

Saphenous nerve

Medial terminal branch of the deep peroneal nerve

Plantar Anatomy

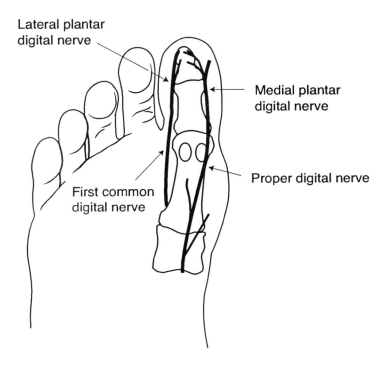

Lateral plantar digital nerve

Medial plantar digital nerve

Proper digital nerve

First common digital nerve

Mayo Block Injections

The Mayo block involves four sticks, a total of approximately 8 mL is used:

1. From dorsomedial to plantar-medial.
2. From dorsomedial to dorsolateral
3. From dorsolateral to plantar-lateral
4. From plantar-medial to plantar-lateral

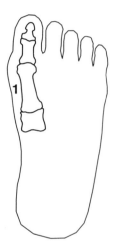

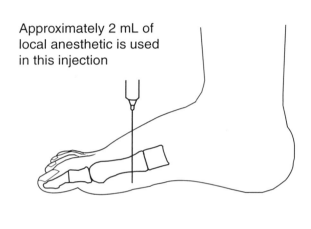

Approximately 2 mL of local anesthetic is used in this injection

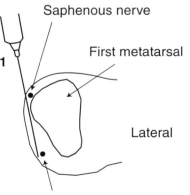

Saphenous nerve

First metatarsal

Trick: This injection is closer to bone than to skin

Medial

Lateral

Proper digital nerve

Approximately 2 mL of local anesthetic is used in this injection

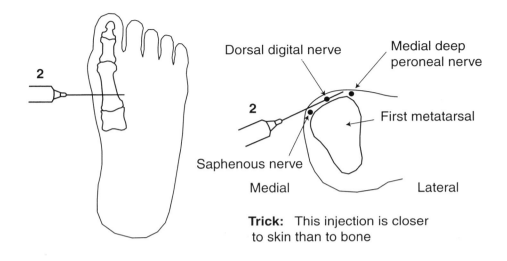

Dorsal digital nerve

Medial deep peroneal nerve

2

First metatarsal

Saphenous nerve

Medial

Lateral

Trick: This injection is closer to skin than to bone

Approximately 2 mL of local anesthetic is used in this injection

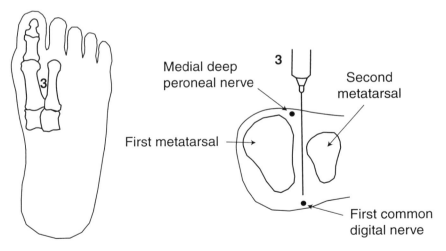

Medial deep peroneal nerve

3

Second metatarsal

First metatarsal

First common digital nerve

Trick: This injection is closer to skin than to bone

Approximately 2 mL of local anesthetic is used in this injection

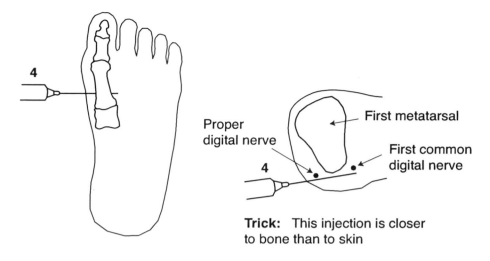

Proper
digital nerve

First metatarsal

First common
digital nerve

Trick: This injection is closer
to bone than to skin

Chapter 4
Sensory Testing of the Foot and Ankle

Frederick G. Lippert III, M.D.

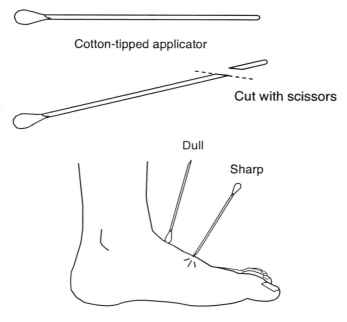

Cotton-tipped applicator

Cut with scissors

Dull

Sharp

Sensory testing of local anesthesia

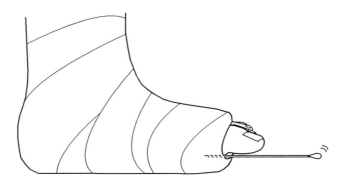

Postoperative sensory testing inside cast

Chapter 5
Assessing Hindfoot Alignment

Frederick G. Lippert III, M.D.
Sigvard T. Hansen Jr., M.D.

Goal: To reach 5° to 7° hindfoot valgus while weightbearing

Standing: Early Predictor of Problems

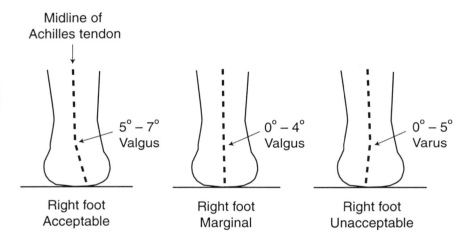

Midline of
Achilles tendon

5° – 7°
Valgus

Right foot
Acceptable

0° – 4°
Valgus

Right foot
Marginal

0° – 5°
Varus

Right foot
Unacceptable

Walking Midstance: Most Critical—No Rollout

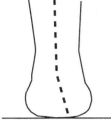 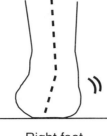

Rollout caused by varus hindfoot alignment, weak peroneals, and stretched lateral ankle ligaments

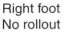

Right foot   Right foot
No rollout   Rollout

Pitfall: Attempt to control with lateral heel wedge torques ipsilateral knee joint

Tricks:
1. Valgus calcaneal osteotomy
2. Peroneus longus to peroneus brevis
3. Split lateral anterior tibial transfer (SPLATT) procedure to lateral foot
4. Brostrom: lateral ankle ligament reconstruction

Evaluating Nonweightbearing Alignment in the Operating Room

Pitfalls: Foot plantar flexed or forefoot not in neutral postion may cause inaccurate reading

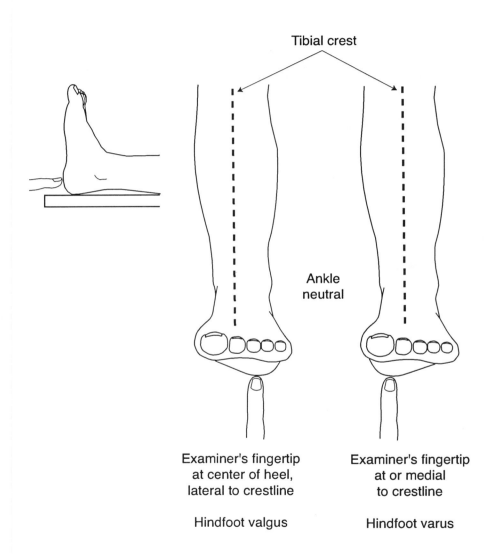

Tibial crest

Ankle neutral

Examiner's fingertip at center of heel, lateral to crestline

Hindfoot valgus

Examiner's fingertip at or medial to crestline

Hindfoot varus

Simulated Weightbearing in the Operating Room

Should feel stable with no wobble

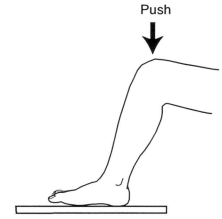

Push

Simulated weightbearing X-ray

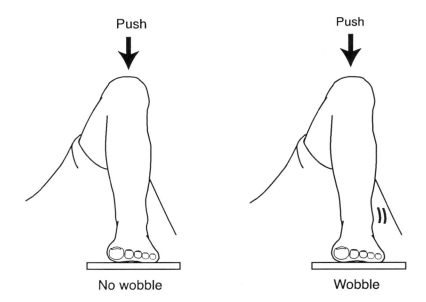

Push	Push
No wobble	Wobble
Hindfoot valgus	Possible hindfoot varus

Nonweightbearing Alignment in the Operating Room

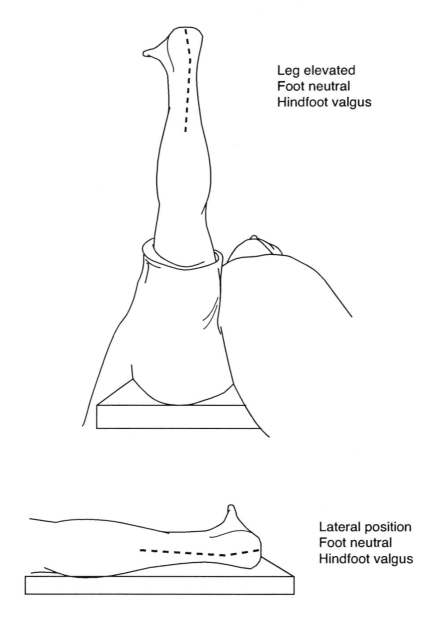

Leg elevated
Foot neutral
Hindfoot valgus

Lateral position
Foot neutral
Hindfoot valgus

Chapter 6 Passing Tendons through Bone Using a Penrose Drain

Edward S. Holt, M.D.

Passing the Tendon through Bone

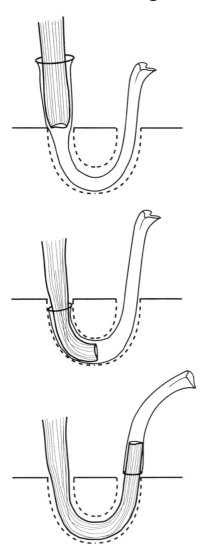

Trick: Let the end of the tendon dry out by wrapping it in dry gauze for 10 to 20 minutes

Trick: Use a 1/4-inch Penrose drain as a passer. Insert 4 to 6 cm of tendon into the Penrose. Pass the other end of the Penrose through the hole and use it to pull the tendon through

Pitfall: The Penrose can be torn by sharp bone spikes, which will leave pieces of drain in the bone tunnel

Trick: Pull the tendon back out and pass a 4- X 4-inch gauze sponge through the hole several times and it will retrieve the pieces of Penrose. Then smooth the sharp spikes and start over

Chapter 7 Passing Tendons through Bone Using a Wire Loop

Frederick G. Lippert III, M.D.
Sigvard T. Hansen Jr., M.D.

Passing the Tendon through Bone
Alternative Method

Trick: To enhance incorporation of the tendon into the bone tunnel, remove the tenosynovium from the tendon with a scalpel

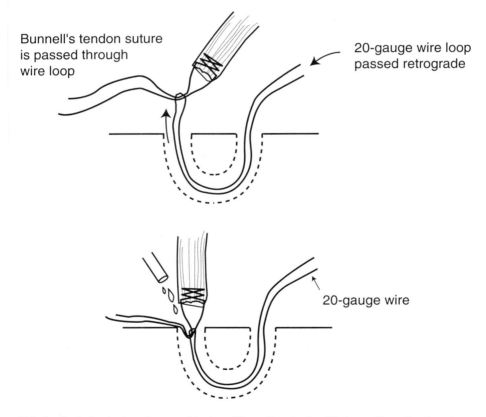

Bunnell's tendon suture is passed through wire loop

20-gauge wire loop passed retrograde

20-gauge wire

Trick: Lubricate tendon and hole with saline to facilitate pulling the tendon through the hole

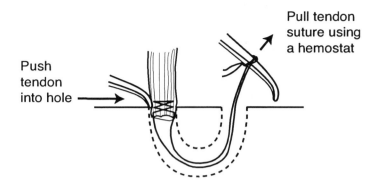

Push
tendon
into hole →

Pull tendon
suture using
a hemostat

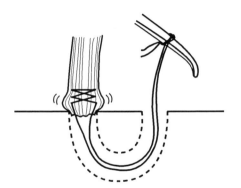

Pitfall: End of the tendon
buckles and impacts

Bail Out:
1. Remove the tendon, taper
   the end, and try again
2. Replace suture

Chapter 8 Obtaining Bone Graft from the Lateral Calcaneus

Frederick G. Lippert III, M.D.
Sigvard T. Hansen Jr., M.D.

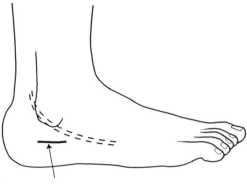

Incision below and slightly posterior to the lateral malleolis

Incision below peroneal tendons

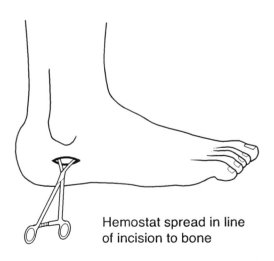

Hemostat spread in line of incision to bone

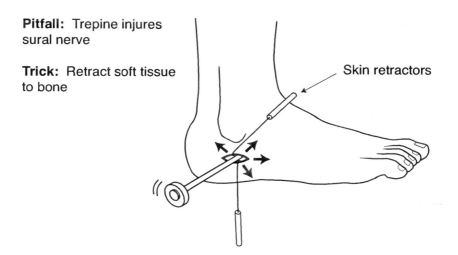

Pitfall: Trepine injures sural nerve

Trick: Retract soft tissue to bone

Skin retractors

Trepine pushed in multiple directions for maximum yield of bone graft

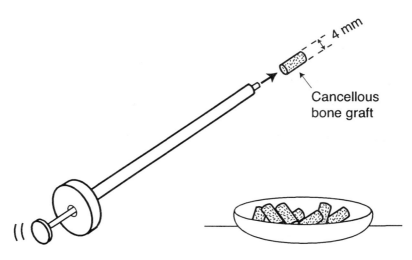

4 mm

Cancellous bone graft

Collect five to seven plugs
Graft ready for placement

Strain-Relieving Bone Graft Technique

Problem: Nonunion from micromotion
Trick: Create spot weld across the interface, which initiates union

Pitfall: Sural nerve wraps around rotating burr
Trick: Use two hands on burr, hold burr perpendicular to bone, retract soft tissue

Pitfall: Destabilizing construct from too many or too large a bone graft site

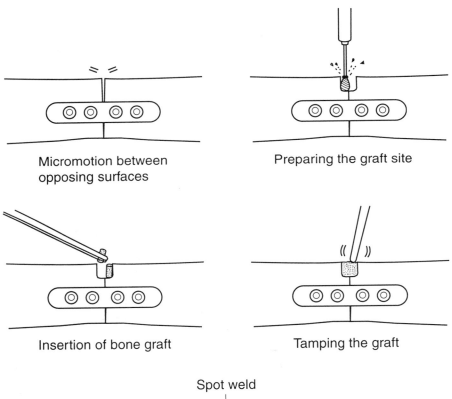

Micromotion between opposing surfaces

Preparing the graft site

Insertion of bone graft

Tamping the graft

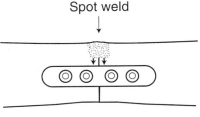

Spot weld

Union propagates from spot weld

Chapter 9
Percutaneous Plantar Fasciotomy

Thomas Franchini, D.P.M.
Frederick G. Lippert III, M.D.

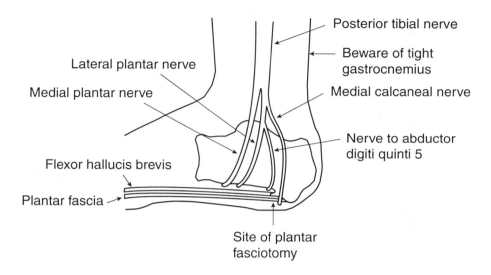

Posterior tibial nerve

Beware of tight gastrocnemius

Lateral plantar nerve

Medial plantar nerve

Medial calcaneal nerve

Nerve to abductor digiti quinti 5

Flexor hallucis brevis

Plantar fascia

Site of plantar fasciotomy

Pitfall: Tight heel cord stretches plantar fascia

Trick: Perform gastrocnemius slide or heel cord release at the same time

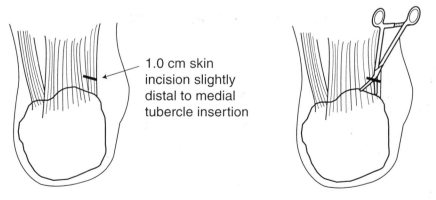

1.0 cm skin incision slightly distal to medial tubercle insertion

Spread soft tissue down to plantar fascia with a hemostat

Assessing Plantar Fascia Borders before Release

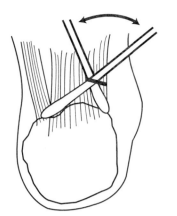

Pitfall: Inaccurate identification of the medial border of the plantar fascia

Trick: Insert a Freer elevator through the skin incision to palpate medial and lateral edges of the plantar fascia

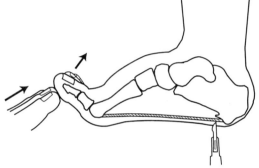

Trick: Tensioning the plantar fascia before medial release accentuates the medial border and facilitates accurate placement of the cut

Releasing the Plantar Fascia

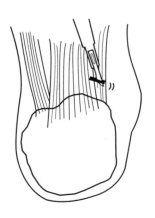

Trick: Insert a no. 15 blade through the skin incision and feel the tensioned medial edge of the plantar fascia, then release the medial one third

Pitfall: Injury to calcaneal nerve or nerve to abductor digiti quinti 5

Trick: Follow landmarks. Cut perpendicular to fascia, which is parallel to the nerves

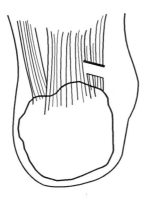

Completed medial one third plantar fascia release

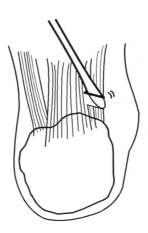

Palpate the extent and completeness of release with a Freer elevator

Chapter 10
Chevron Bunionectomy

Frederick G. Lippert III, M.D.
Sigvard T. Hansen Jr., M.D.

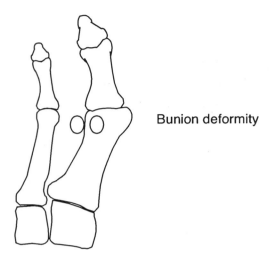

Bunion deformity

Capsular release

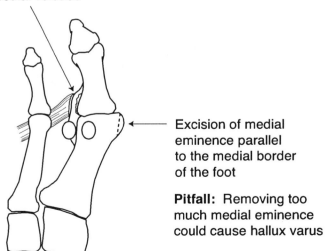

Excision of medial
eminence parallel
to the medial border
of the foot

Pitfall: Removing too
much medial eminence
could cause hallux varus

Using a Guide Wire to Determine the Plane of the Osteotomy

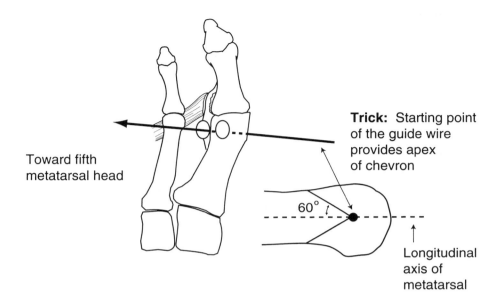

Toward fifth
metatarsal head

Trick: Starting point
of the guide wire
provides apex
of chevron

60°

Longitudinal
axis of
metatarsal

The Effect of the Guide Wire Placement on the Inclination of the Osteotomy Plane

Trick: Inclination of the guide wire determines the position of the metarsal head in the coronal plane

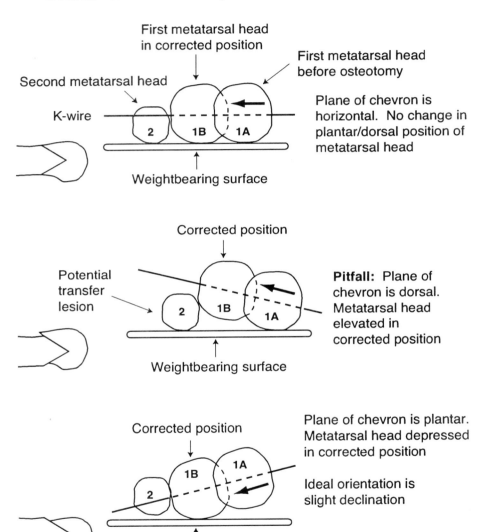

First metatarsal head in corrected position

First metatarsal head before osteotomy

Second metatarsal head

K-wire

Plane of chevron is horizontal. No change in plantar/dorsal position of metatarsal head

2   1B   1A

Weightbearing surface

Corrected position

Potential transfer lesion

Pitfall: Plane of chevron is dorsal. Metatarsal head elevated in corrected position

2   1B   1A

Weightbearing surface

Plane of chevron is plantar. Metatarsal head depressed in corrected position

Corrected position

Ideal orientation is slight declination

1A   1B   2

Weightbearing surface

Maintaining Saw Blade Alignment

Trick: Surgeon maintains the saw blade in line with the guide wire

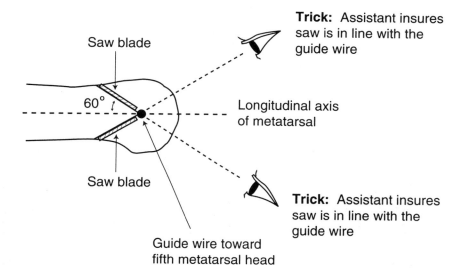

Trick: Assistant insures saw is in line with the guide wire

Saw blade

Longitudinal axis of metatarsal

60°

Saw blade

Trick: Assistant insures saw is in line with the guide wire

Guide wire toward fifth metatarsal head

Translating the Metatarsal Head to the Corrected Position

Head translated laterally but still in valgus alignment

Trick: Head impacted medially to correct valgus alignment

Completed chevron bunionectomy

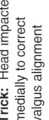

Guide wire

Osteotomy

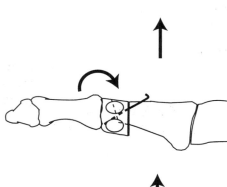

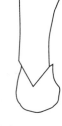

Criteria of Acceptability:
1. Bunion deformity is corrected
2. Distal metatarsal articular angle is corrected
3. Metatarsal head is positioned over sesamoids
4. There is a slight declination of the metatarsal head
5. Pin fixation is achieved

Pitfall: Impaction of hallux against the second toe after chevron bunionectomy due to hallux valgus interphalangeus

Tricks: Perform medial closing wedge osteotomy (Akin) and/or rotate capital segment into slight varus and impact it

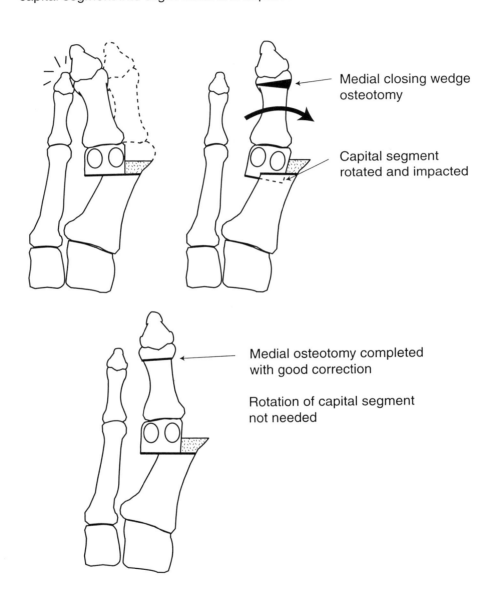

Medial closing wedge osteotomy

Capital segment rotated and impacted

Medial osteotomy completed with good correction

Rotation of capital segment not needed

Chapter 11
Closing Wedge Bunionectomy

Frederick G. Lippert III, M.D.
Sigvard T. Hansen Jr., M.D.

Handling the Medial Eminence

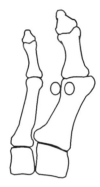

Excision   Recontouring

Pitfall: Excessive resection, tibial sesamoid uncovered, hallux varus

Oblique Closing Wedge

Capsular release only if needed after correction

Pitfall: Hallux varus

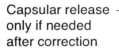

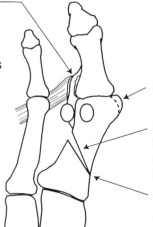

Recontour medial eminence

Laterally based closing wedge osteotomy; adjust cut until desired correction is achieved

Trick: Preserve apex and periosteal hinge for stability

Transverse Closing Wedge
Alternative Osteotomy Position

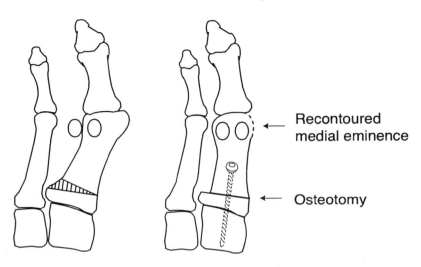

← Recontoured medial eminence

← Osteotomy

Fixation of the Closing Wedge Osteotomy

Trick: Place proximal screw first. Rotate distal segment to maintain weightbearing parabola, then place distal screw

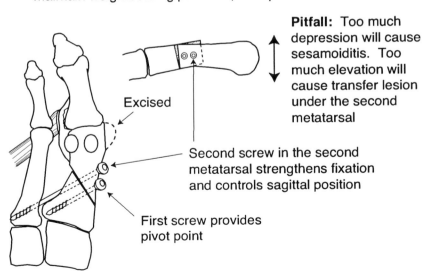

Pitfall: Too much depression will cause sesamoiditis. Too much elevation will cause transfer lesion under the second metatarsal

Excised

Second screw in the second metatarsal strengthens fixation and controls sagittal position

First screw provides pivot point

Chapter 12 Scarf Bunionectomy

Craig Williams, D.P.M., D.A.B.P.S.

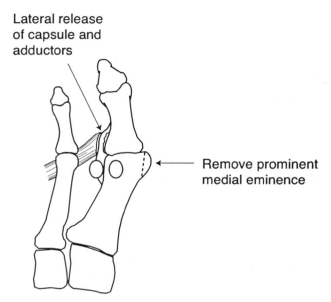

Lateral release of capsule and adductors

Remove prominent medial eminence

Classic Scarf

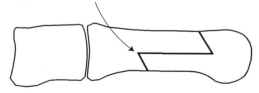

Pitfall: Potential for stress rises at this point

Pitfall: Proximal plantar cut is difficult to see and access through dorsal incision

Pitfall: Making the two cuts too perpendicular to long axis of first metatarsal (losing stability of this osteotomy)

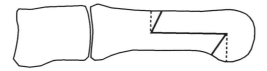

Trick: Reverse cuts. Making the plantar cut distal (can be the same as a chevron cut) makes it easier to retract skin to access the plantar cut and allows complete visualization of dorsal proximal cut

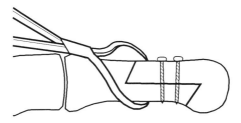

Trick: Stabilization with bone clamp prior to screw fixation. Use a reduction clamp to hold bone stable while placing fixation

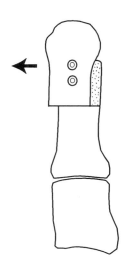 Like a chevron osteotomy, it may be necessary to release lateral soft tissue to allow the capital fragment to slide over laterally

Capital fragment

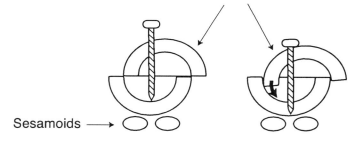

Sesamoids ⟶

Pitfall: If the capital fragment is too far lateral, it will trough into the medullary canal when screws are tightened

Trick: Rotate the capital fragment enough to engage the cortices

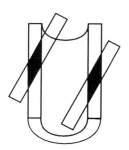

Correcting the Distal Metatarsal Articular Angle

Pitfall: Bunion is corrected but DMAA is still facing laterally

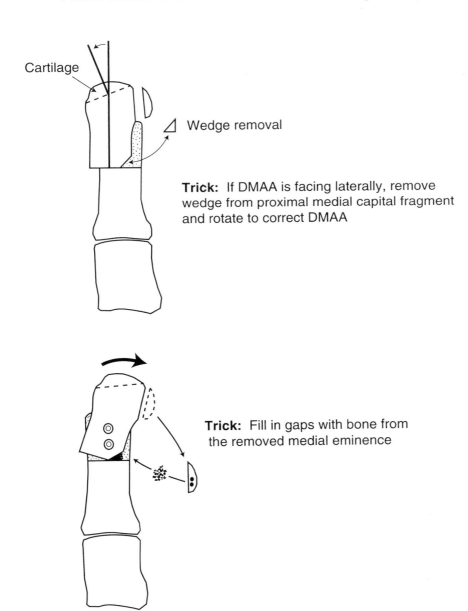

Cartilage

Wedge removal

Trick: If DMAA is facing laterally, remove wedge from proximal medial capital fragment and rotate to correct DMAA

Trick: Fill in gaps with bone from the removed medial eminence

Chapter 13 Lapidus Bunionectomy

Sigvard T. Hansen Jr., M.D.
Frederick G. Lippert III, M.D.

Osteotomies of the Lapidus Bunionectomy

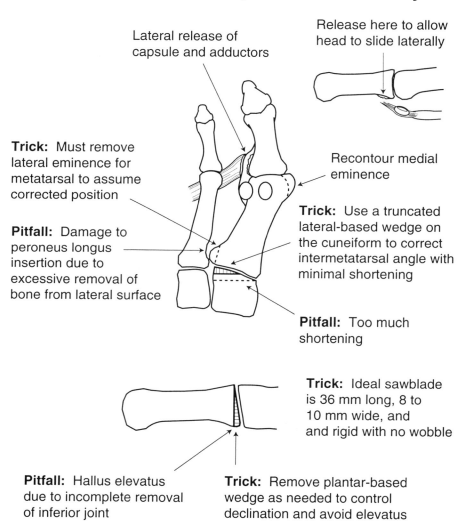

Lateral release of capsule and adductors

Release here to allow head to slide laterally

Trick: Must remove lateral eminence for metatarsal to assume corrected position

Recontour medial eminence

Trick: Use a truncated lateral-based wedge on the cuneiform to correct intermetatarsal angle with minimal shortening

Pitfall: Damage to peroneus longus insertion due to excessive removal of bone from lateral surface

Pitfall: Too much shortening

Trick: Ideal sawblade is 36 mm long, 8 to 10 mm wide, and and rigid with no wobble

Pitfall: Hallus elevatus due to incomplete removal of inferior joint

Trick: Remove plantar-based wedge as needed to control declination and avoid elevatus

Stabilization of Construct before Fixation

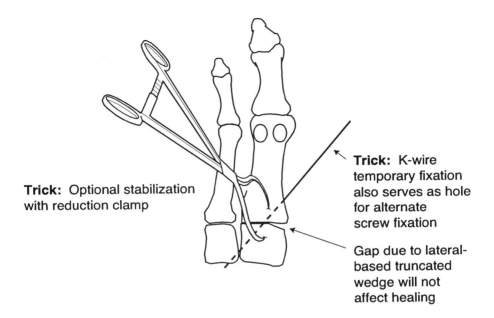

Trick: Optional stabilization with reduction clamp

Trick: K-wire temporary fixation also serves as hole for alternate screw fixation

Gap due to lateral-based truncated wedge will not affect healing

Screw Placement

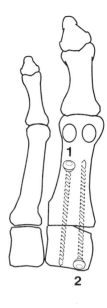

Trick: Start screw no. 1 (3.5 mm cortical screw) at midshaft to obtain best mechanical advantage

Trick: Use long 2.5 mm drill bit to avoid drill chuck chafing skin

Trick: Start screw no. 2 (3.5 mm cortical screw) in subchondral bone. Parallel screw pattern provides maximum rigidity

Notched dorsal cortex provides recess for screw head

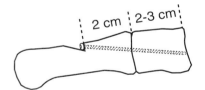

2 cm ┊ 2-3 cm┊

Average total screw length is 45 to 50 mm

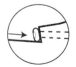

Trick: Correct pathway, screw moves parallel to floor of notch and engages vertical face

Pitfall: Incorrect pathway, screw impacts floor of notch and is levered dorsally, fracturing the cortex

The Shear Strain–Relieving Bone Graft

Trick: The shear strain–relieving bone graft enhances union by increasing the surface area

Trick: Obtain graft using bone biopsy trepine

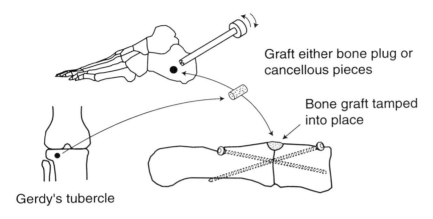

Graft either bone plug or cancellous pieces

Bone graft tamped into place

Gerdy's tubercle

The Completed Lapidus Bunionectomy

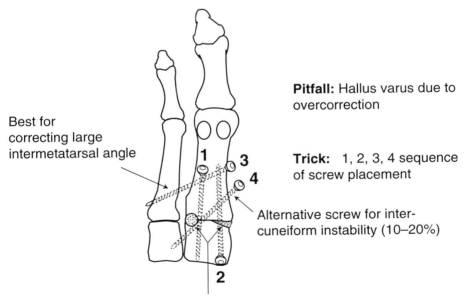

Best for correcting large intermetatarsal angle

Pitfall: Hallus varus due to overcorrection

Trick: 1, 2, 3, 4 sequence of screw placement

Alternative screw for inter-cuneiform instability (10–20%)

Trick: Shear strain–relieving bone grafts

Lengthening and/or Plantar Flexing the Hallux as Part of the Lapidus Bunionectomy

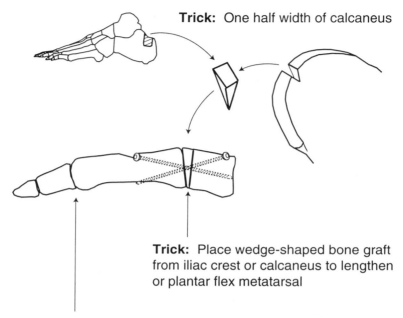

Trick: One half width of calcaneus

Trick: Place wedge-shaped bone graft from iliac crest or calcaneus to lengthen or plantar flex metatarsal

Pitfall: Too much lengthening when MTP joint is stiff from prior surgery will decrease ROM

Trick: Shorten second metatarsal instead

Chapter 14 Hallux Varus

Frederick G. Lippert III, M.D.
Sigvard T. Hansen Jr., M.D.

Primary Causes and Treatment

1. Excessive resection of the medial eminence
2. Overcorrection of the bunion causing a negative intermetatarsal angle
3. Removal of lateral sesamoid
4. Tendon imbalance and contracture perpetuating deformity
5. Multiple, simultaneous bunionectomy procedures

Excessive Resection of the Medial Eminence

Goals:

1. Release medial MTP joint capsular contractures
2. Correct alignment
3. Balance tendon forces

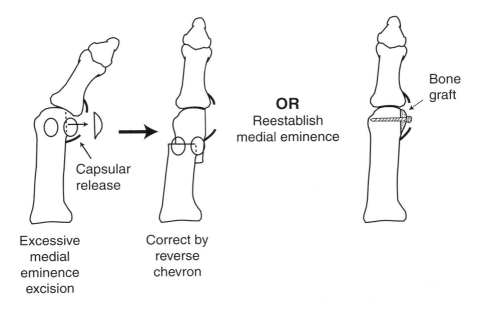

Capsular release

OR

Reestablish medial eminence

Bone graft

Excessive medial eminence excision

Correct by reverse chevron

Overcorrection Causes Negative Intermetatarsal Angle

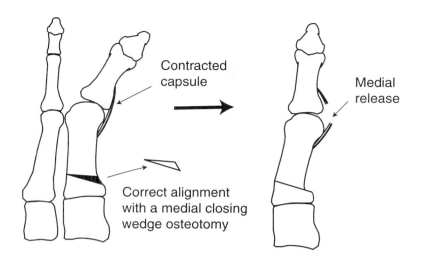

Contracted capsule

Correct alignment with a medial closing wedge osteotomy

Medial release

Removal of Lateral Sesamoid

Tendon Imbalance

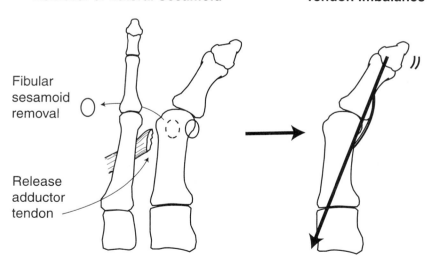

Fibular sesamoid removal

Release adductor tendon

Pitfall: Adduction deformity of lesser toes results

Pitfall: Medialized tendon vector perpetuates deformity

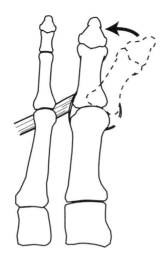

Reattach adductor tendon
to lateral capsule

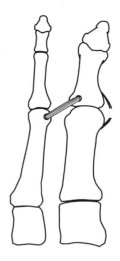

Using lesser toe
extensor tendon

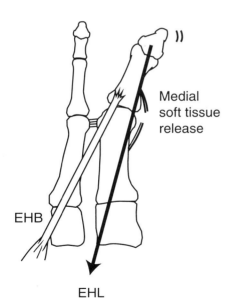

Medial
soft tissue
release

EHB

EHL

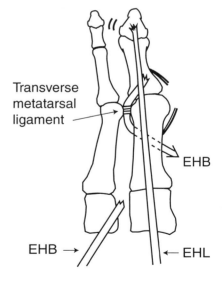

Transverse
metatarsal
ligament

EHB

EHB →

← EHL

Using distal EHB tendon

Correction of Tendon Imbalance by Changing Line of Tendon Action

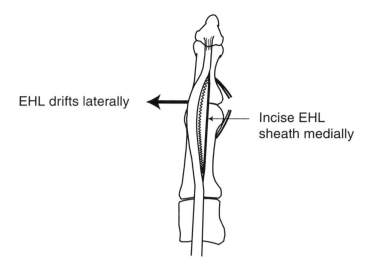

EHL drifts laterally

Incise EHL
sheath medially

Correction of Tendon Imbalance by Lateralizing the Extensor Hallucis Longus

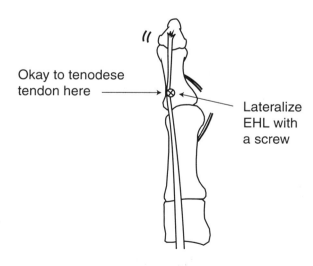

Okay to tenodese
tendon here

Lateralize
EHL with
a screw

Correction of Tendon Imbalance by Extensor Hallucis Longus Split Tendon Transfer

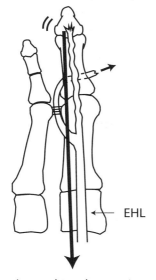

Pitfall: Excessive tightening of EHL transfer will produce slack in the distal EHL tendon, resulting in toe drop

Pitfall: Hallux drifts into varus over time

Trick: Place in slight hallux valgus alignment to lateralize tendon vector

← EHL

Lateral tendon vector
maintains correction

Correction of Tendon Imbalance by Extensor Hallucis Longus Tenodesis with Interphalangeal Joint Fusion

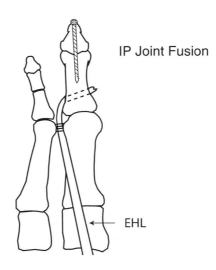

IP Joint Fusion

← EHL

Maintaining Surgical Correction of Hallux Varus

Pitfall: Gradual recurrence

Tricks: Overcorrect and stabilize with a K-wire for 3 to 4 weeks

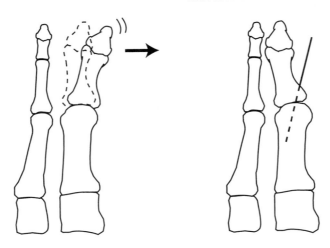

Hallux varus potentiates lesser toe adduction

Additional Options

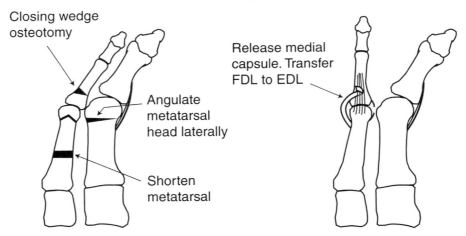

Closing wedge osteotomy

Angulate metatarsal head laterally

Shorten metatarsal

Release medial capsule. Transfer FDL to EDL

Pitfall: Adduction deformity of lesser toes may cause recurrence of or perpetuate hallux varus

Trick: Correct adduction deformity of lesser toes before addressing the hallux varus

Chapter 15
Cheilectomy for Hallux Rigidus

Frederick G. Lippert III, M.D.
Sigvard T. Hansen Jr., M.D.

Alternative skin incisions
of the left first metatarsal

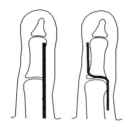

Dorsal osteophytes

Sesamoid adhesions

Pathomechanics

Dorsal spur blocks dorsiflexion

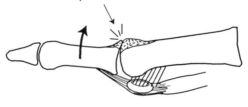

Excision of Osteophytes

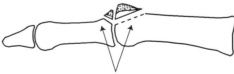

Cheilectomy margins

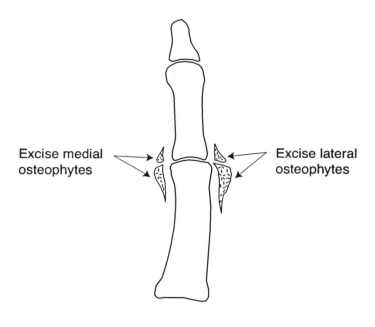

Excise medial osteophytes

Excise lateral osteophytes

Trick: Round off corners

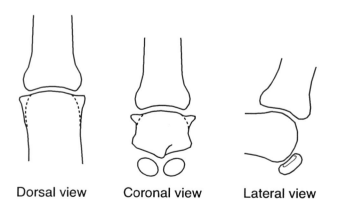

Dorsal view   Coronal view   Lateral view

Trick: Excise phalangeal dorsal osteophyte

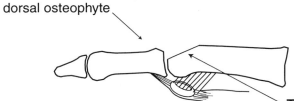

Trick: Excise dorsal osteophyte and dorsal third of metatarsal head

Obtaining Adequate Dorsiflexion

Dorsiflexion without sesamoid adhesions released

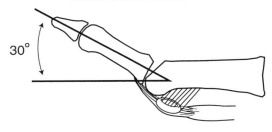

30°

Trick: Sesamoid adhesions released with McGlamry elevator or osteotome

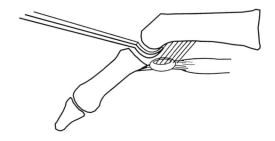

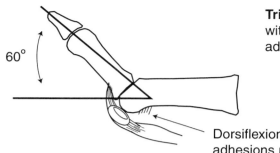

Trick: Inject capsular tissues with steroid to avoid capsular adhesions

60°

Dorsiflexion with sesamoid adhesions released

Trick: Tenodese EHB and EHL to the proximal phalanx

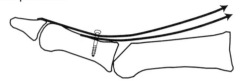

Combined extensor pull forces joint to glide dorsally and not impinge

Alternative Osteotomies to Achieve More Dorsiflexion at the Metatarsal Phalangeal Joint

Dorsiflexion osteotomy   Shortening osteotomy

Reduction of the dorsal prominance of the metatarsal head

Pitfall: Too much dorsiflexion, toe hits top of shoe
Contraindicated with long second metatarsal

Chapter 16 Cock-up Hallux

Sigvard T. Hansen Jr., M.D.
Frederick G. Lippert III, M.D.

Problems:
1. Dorsal subluxation of MTP joint
2. Contracted capsule
3. EHL and FHL perpetuate deformity
4. Metatarsal plantar flexed
5. EHL substitutes for weak TA
6. Stretched FHB causes dorsal subluxation

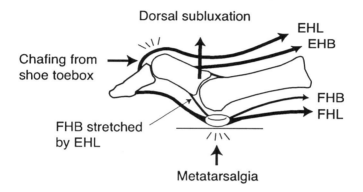

Correction of Cock-up Hallux by Soft Tissue Release and Tendon Transfers

Trick: Weaken EHL by transfer to TA

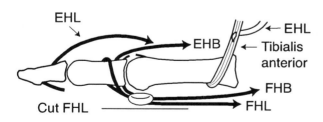

Pitfall: Subcutaneous lump results from suture and tendon transfers

Pitfall: Medial accessory EHL tendon holds toe extended

Trick: Divide tendon if present

Trick: Reduce dorsal subluxation by dorsal capsulotomy and transfer FHL to proximal phalanx

Correction of Cock-up Hallux by Metatarsal Phalangeal Fusion

Trick: Transfer EHL to tibialis anterior or to base of the metatarsal. Fuse MTP joint and tibial sesamoid to metatarsal head

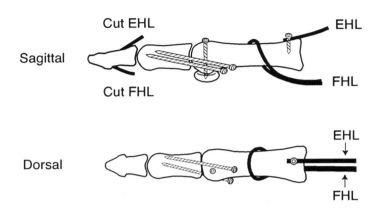

Chapter 17
Metatarsal Phalangeal Fusion

Frederick G. Lippert III, M.D.
Sigvard T. Hansen Jr., M.D.

Concept: Joint contours preserved for maximum surface area stability and flexibility of positioning

Trick: Cartilage is removed to subchondral bone, which is drilled

Trick: Retrograde drilling of glide holes while joint is flexed facilitates placement of screws across each other

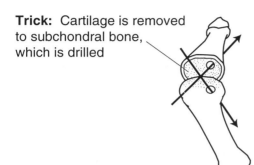

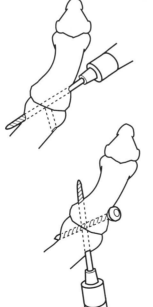

Joint reduced for drilling into metatarsal

MTP joint in final fusion position. Distal 3.5 mm cortical screw in place

Preparation for proximal screw

Completed Fixation

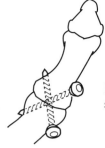

Both screws in place,
solid cortical bite, rigid fixation

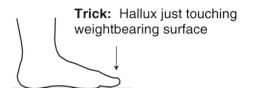

Trick: Hallux just touching
weightbearing surface

Pitfall: Too much dorsiflexion
or plantar flexion

Trick: Simulated weightbearing lateral X-ray

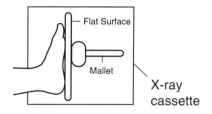

Flat Surface

Mallet

X-ray
cassette

Pitfall: Inadequate fixation

Bail Out:

Two K-wires

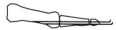

Dorsal plate

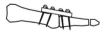

Screw placement

Chapter 18 Tailor's Bunionette

Sigvard T. Hansen Jr., M.D.
Frederick G. Lippert III, M.D.

Types

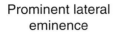

Prominent lateral
eminence

Distal lateral
angulation

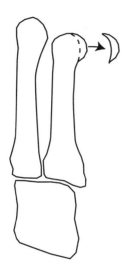

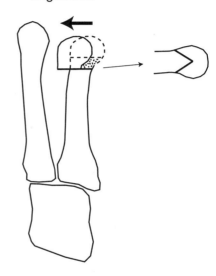

Excise eminence

Medial chevron

Oblique Osteotomy of the Fifth Metatarsal

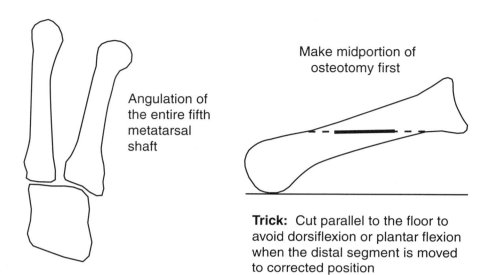

Angulation of the entire fifth metatarsal shaft

Make midportion of osteotomy first

Trick: Cut parallel to the floor to avoid dorsiflexion or plantar flexion when the distal segment is moved to corrected position

Pitfall: Osteotomy too horizontal

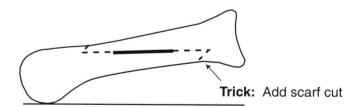

Trick: Add scarf cut

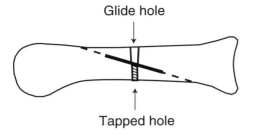

Glide hole

Tapped hole

Pitfalls: Very difficult to drill and tap once osteotomy is completed
1. Thin osteotomy surfaces fracture easily
2. Minimal area for two screws

Trick: Drill glide hole through dorsal cortex and tap far cortex before osteotomy is completed

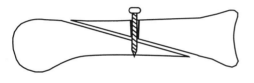

Osteotomy completed with screw in place

Tricks:
1. Insert central screw
2. Complete osteotomy
3. Rotate plantar segment medially

Plantar segment rotated medially around central screw

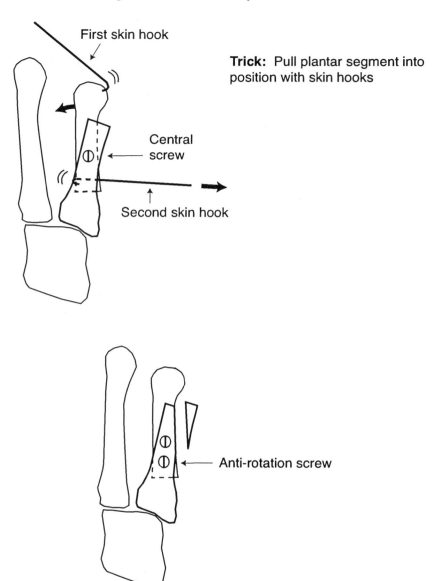

First skin hook

Trick: Pull plantar segment into position with skin hooks

Central screw

Second skin hook

Anti-rotation screw

Chapter 19 Avulsion Fracture Base Proximal Phalanx Hallux

Frederick G. Lippert III, M.D.
Sigvard T. Hansen Jr., M.D.

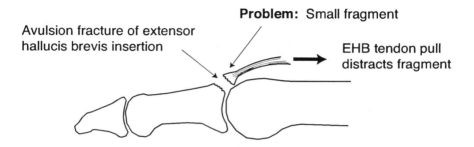

Avulsion fracture of extensor
hallucis brevis insertion

Problem: Small fragment

EHB tendon pull
distracts fragment

Fracture Reduction and Fixation

Trick: K-wire retrograded through fracture site and out the tip of the toe

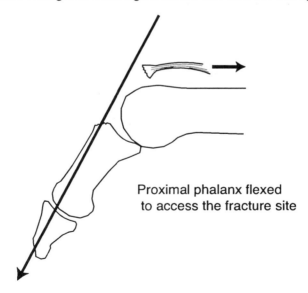

Proximal phalanx flexed
to access the fracture site

Trick: Fracture reduction maneuvers

K-wire just distal
to fracture

2. Push down with thumb to
   reduce fracture

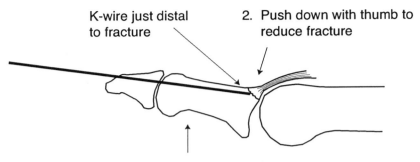

1. Hyperextend distal phalanx
   to decrease EHB distraction force

Completed Reduction and Fixation

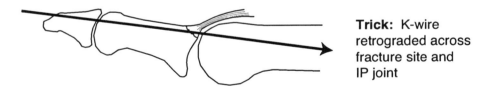

Trick: K-wire
retrograded across
fracture site and
IP joint

Chapter 20 Metatarsal Parabola and Weightbearing Asymmetry

Frederick G. Lippert III, M.D.
Sigvard T. Hansen Jr., M.D.

Etiology
1. Long metatarsal (usually number 2)
2. Plantar-flexed metatarsal

Result
1. Intractable keratoses
2. Metatarsalgia
3. MTP synovitis and capsular laxity
4. Dorsal subluxation of the MTP joint
5. Crossover toe deformity

Pitfall: Metatarsalgia from tight gastrosoleus complex
Trick: Gastrocnemius slide or percutaneous heel cord release

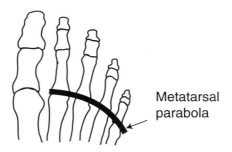

Metatarsal parabola

Ideal relative metatarsal head lengths

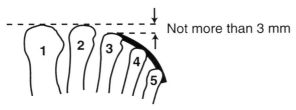

Not more than 3 mm

Pitfalls:
No. 2 too long, metatarsalgia under metatarsal 2
No. 2 too short, transfer lesion under metatarsal 3

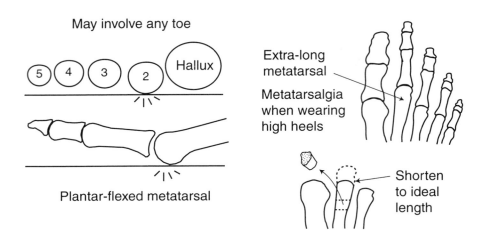

May involve any toe

5 4 3 2 Hallux

Plantar-flexed metatarsal

Extra-long metatarsal

Metatarsalgia when wearing high heels

Shorten to ideal length

Methods of Shortening the Long Metatarsal

Tricks:
1. Attach plate to proximal segment first
2. Clamp distal segment and complete fixation with dynamic compression plate technique

Partial Diaphysectomy

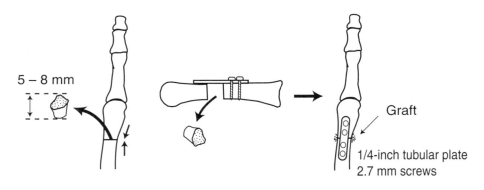

5 – 8 mm

Graft

1/4-inch tubular plate
2.7 mm screws

Pitfall: Excessive shortening
Trick: Leave first and second metatarsals longer than third

Weil Osteotomy

Pitfall: Osteotomy plane not parallel to weightbearing surface causes declination of the capital segment

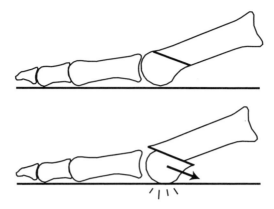

Trick: Osteotomy made parallel to weightbearing surface

Desired cut

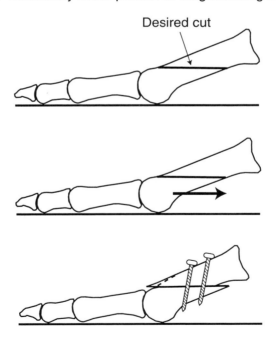

Methods of Elevating the Plantar-flexed Metatarsal

Pitfall: All four osteotomies can cause excessive elevation and transfer lesions

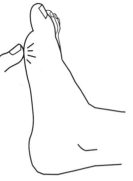

Trick: Palpate metatarsal head presentation for symmetry before fixing final position

Sliding Oblique Osteotomy

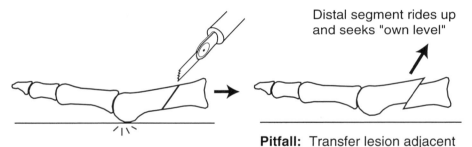

Distal segment rides up and seeks "own level"

Pitfall: Transfer lesion adjacent to metatarsal heads

Vertical Chevron Osteotomy

Trick: Control position of the metatarsal head with a pin

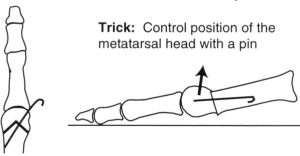

Plantar Condylectomy

Trick: Best for keel-like plantar condyle as seen on sesamoid view

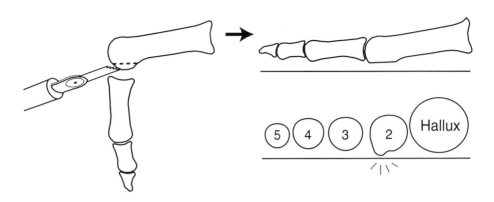

Dorsal Closing Wedge Osteotomy

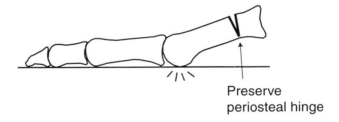

Preserve
periosteal hinge

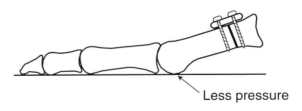

Less pressure

Chapter 21 Lesser Toe Deformities

Frederick G. Lippert III, M.D.
Sigvard T. Hansen Jr., M.D.

Problems of the Fixed Toe Deformity

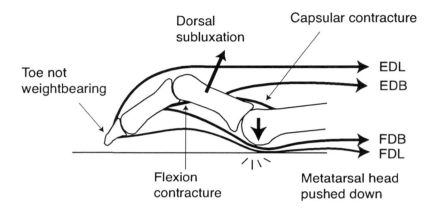

Treatment of Fixed Lesser Toe Deformity

Goals:

1. Reduce dorsal subluxation of MTP joint
2. Restore flexion power of lesser toe
3. Correct length and flexion contractures through PIP joint

Sequence of Release:

1. EDL
2. EDB
3. Dorsal capsule

Trick: Let EDL proximal to toes 2 to 4 retract.
Transfer EDL no. 5 to the peroneus tertius

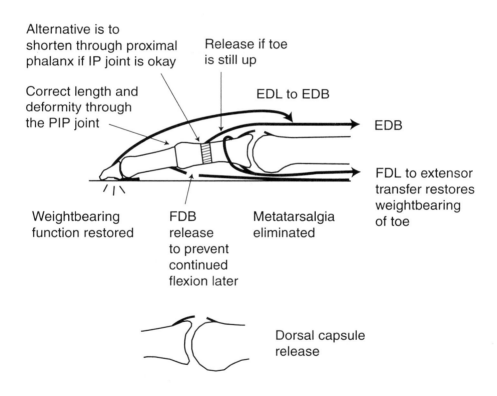

Alternative is to shorten through proximal phalanx if IP joint is okay

Release if toe is still up

Correct length and deformity through the PIP joint

EDL to EDB

EDB

FDL to extensor transfer restores weightbearing of toe

Weightbearing function restored

FDB release to prevent continued flexion later

Metatarsalgia eliminated

Dorsal capsule release

Girdlestone-Taylor Procedure
for Fixed Toe Deformities

Dorsal incision

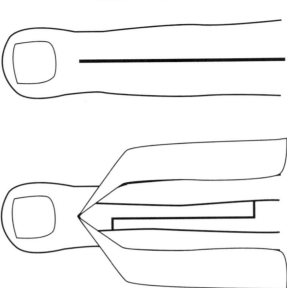

Trick: EDL Z-plasty for exposure of PIP joint and extensor contracture release

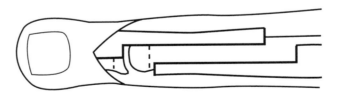

Trick: PIP joint resection corrects deformity and adjusts length

Plantar plate incision

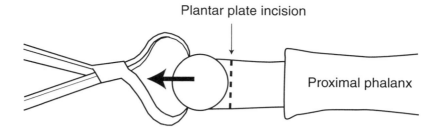

Proximal phalanx

Trick: Flex toe at PIP joint; pulling with towel clip provides stability

Release FDL distally

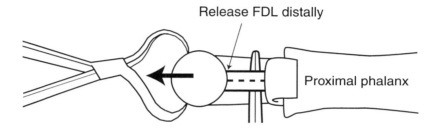

Proximal phalanx

Locate FDL between FDB

FDL split along median raphe

FDL

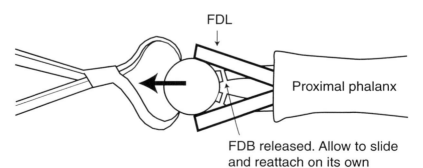

Proximal phalanx

FDB released. Allow to slide
and reattach on its own

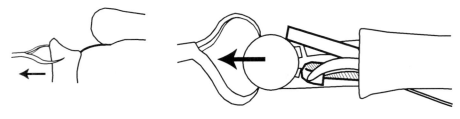

FDL pulled proximally

Trick: Retrieve FDL slips with hemostat. Grab distal end of tendon and deliver it proximally.

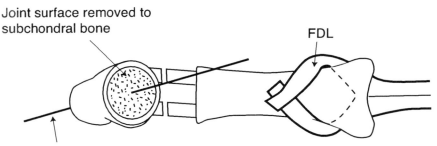

Joint surface removed to subchondral bone

FDL

Pin passed retrograde, then antegrade for fixation

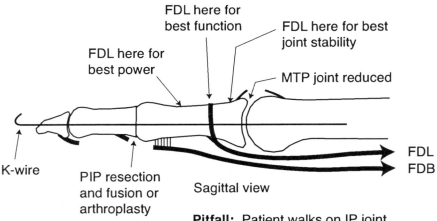

FDL here for best function

FDL here for best joint stability

FDL here for best power

MTP joint reduced

K-wire

PIP resection and fusion or arthroplasty

Sagittal view

FDL
FDB

Pitfall: Patient walks on IP joint
Trick: Tighten FDL when ankle is at 90°

Crossover Toe

Goals: Correct dynamic and static deformity, restore medial/lateral balance, and maintain toe flexion power

Overloaded second MTP joint
Synovitis
Capsular laxity

Trick: Shorten metatarsal to balance capsule tension, reduce second MTP joint overload and prevent traumatic synovitis

Contracted capsule

Cortical thickening due to overload

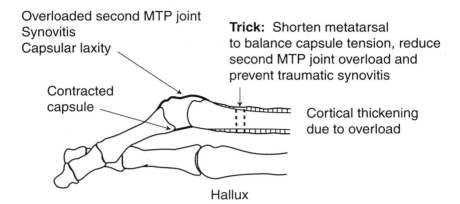

Hallux

Pitfall: Tendons perpetuate deformity

Trick: Restore alignment and balance tendon forces by FDL to proximal phalanx transfer

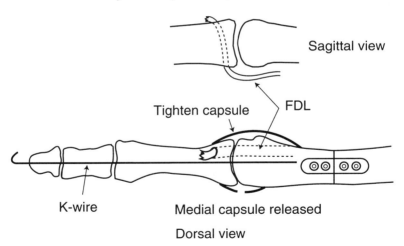

Sagittal view

Tighten capsule   FDL

K-wire   Medial capsule released

Dorsal view

Tricks:
1. Rebalance weight under first and second metatarsal heads
2. Shorten second metatarsal if longer than first
3. Intrinsicplasty—flexor to extensor transfer

Static Claw Toe Deformity with
Flexor Digitorum Longus Contracture

Goals:
1. Identify the underlying cause
2. Restore toe alignment and eliminate clawing

Pitfall: Releasing FDL at medial malleolus may not address FDL and FHL tether to distal tibial fracture or deep posterior compartment syndrome.

Trick: Release FDL and FDB tendons at PIP joint with contractures secondary to posterior compartment syndrome. Check lesser toe flexion with ankle in plantarflexion and dorsiflexion

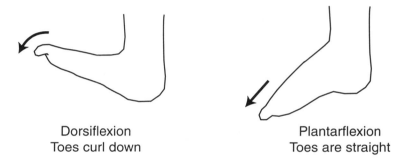

Dorsiflexion
Toes curl down

Plantarflexion
Toes are straight

Midlateral incision

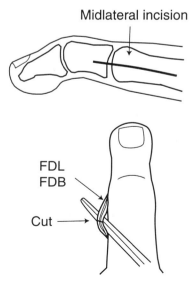

FDL
FDB

Cut →

Dynamic Claw Deformity without Flexor Digitorum Longus Contracture

The Flexor to Extensor Intrinsicplasty

Goals:
1. Eliminate claw deformity
2. Restore normal toe alignment
3. Maintain toe flexion power
4. Maintain a supple toe

Pitfall: FDL too tight and drives PIP joint into floor

Trick: Tension with ankle at 90^0

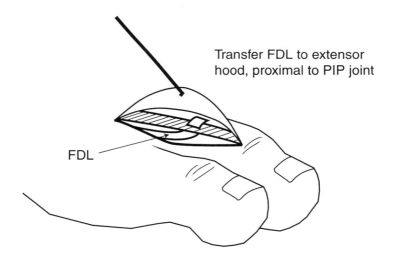

Transfer FDL to extensor hood, proximal to PIP joint

FDL

Pitfall: Excessive toe length with PIP contracture

Trick: Intrinsicplasty plus PIP resection and fusion or arthroplasty

Dynamic Alternative to Interphalangeal Resection
Fusion of Claw Toes

Problems: Tight Achilles' tendon, weak tibialis anterior, hyperactive lesser toe extensors

Pitfall: EDL reattaches through intact sheath
Trick: Excise sheath

Pitfall: Doing procedure without correcting tight Achilles' tendon

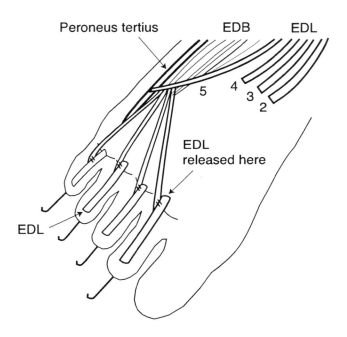

Sequence of release:
1. EDL
2. EDB
3. Dorsal capsule

Tricks:
1. Release EDL proximal to MTP joints
2. Release MTP joint capsular as needed
3. Transfer EDL slip 5 to peroneus tertius
4. Let EDL slips 2 through 4 retract
5. Attach distal EDL cut ends to EDB slips
6. Hold in corrected position with K-wire as required

Chapter 22 Calcaneal Osteotomies

Frederick G. Lippert III, M.D.
Sigvard T. Hansen Jr., M.D.

Osteotomy Placement

Oblique osteotomy corrects medial lateral hindfoot deformity

Osteotomized tubercle must contain:
1. Origin of the plantar fascia
2. Weightbearing surface
3. Insertion of the Achilles' tendon

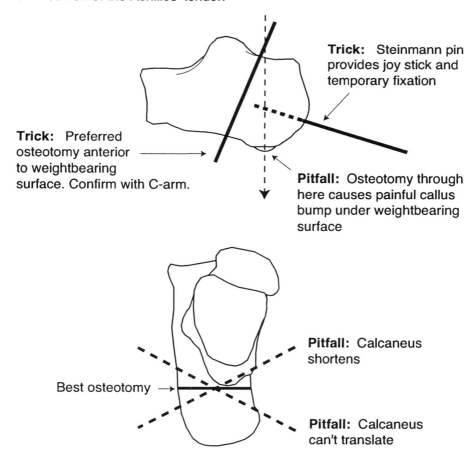

Trick: Steinmann pin provides joy stick and temporary fixation

Trick: Preferred osteotomy anterior to weightbearing surface. Confirm with C-arm.

Pitfall: Osteotomy through here causes painful callus bump under weightbearing surface

Pitfall: Calcaneus shortens

Best osteotomy →

Pitfall: Calcaneus can't translate

Screw Placement

Trick: Place screw for best bone purchase

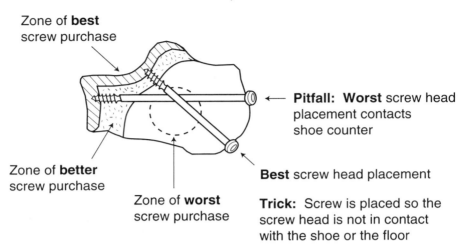

Zone of **best** screw purchase

Pitfall: Worst screw head placement contacts shoe counter

Zone of **better** screw purchase

Zone of **worst** screw purchase

Best screw head placement

Trick: Screw is placed so the screw head is not in contact with the shoe or the floor

Vertical Osteotomy Adjusts Calcaneal Height

Indications: Alternative to the distraction bone block osteotomy

Osteotomy line →

Trick: To depress calcaneus, position osteotomy line vertically, behind posterior facet and anterior to weightbearing surface

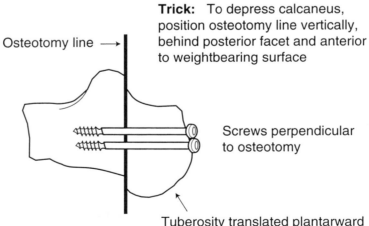

Screws perpendicular to osteotomy

Tuberosity translated plantarward

Varus and Valgus Osteotomies

Calcaneal osteotomy used for start of translational varus and valgus osteotomies

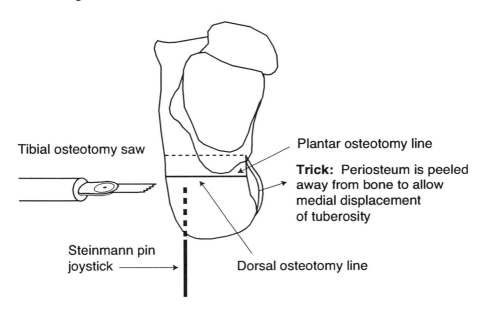

Tibial osteotomy saw

Plantar osteotomy line

Trick: Periosteum is peeled away from bone to allow medial displacement of tuberosity

Steinmann pin joystick ⟶

Dorsal osteotomy line

Trick: Use curved AO elevator to free periosteum on the medial side

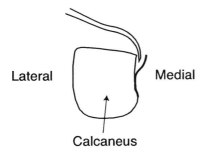

Lateral

Medial

Calcaneus

Trick: Distract periosteum with lamina spreader
1. Start with toothless small spreader
2. Switch to long handle, wide blade, small teeth spreader

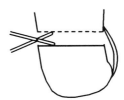

Screw pattern for translational varus osteotomy

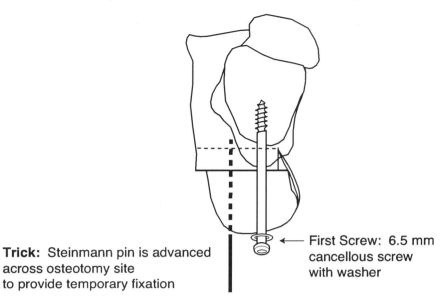

Trick: Steinmann pin is advanced across osteotomy site to provide temporary fixation

First Screw: 6.5 mm cancellous screw with washer

Completed translational varus osteotomy

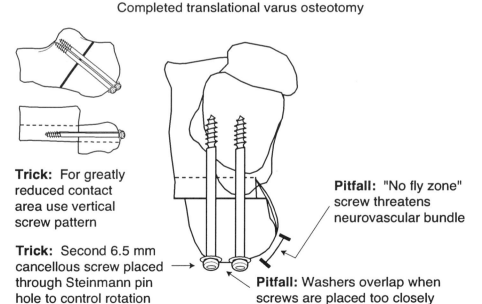

Trick: For greatly reduced contact area use vertical screw pattern

Trick: Second 6.5 mm cancellous screw placed through Steinmann pin hole to control rotation

Pitfall: "No fly zone" screw threatens neurovascular bundle

Pitfall: Washers overlap when screws are placed too closely

Translational Valgus Osteotomy

Screw pattern

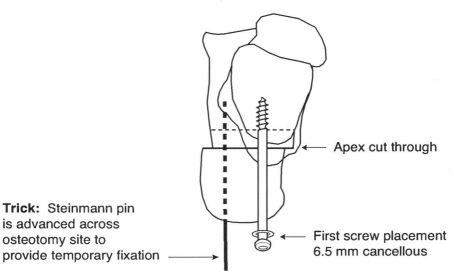

Trick: Steinmann pin is advanced across osteotomy site to provide temporary fixation →

← Apex cut through

← First screw placement 6.5 mm cancellous

Completed translational valgus osteotomy

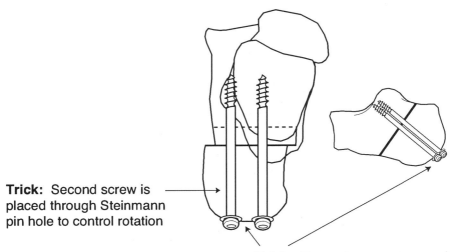

Trick: Second screw is placed through Steinmann pin hole to control rotation →

Trick: Separate screws enough to prevent overlap of washers

Valgus Closing Wedge Osteotomy

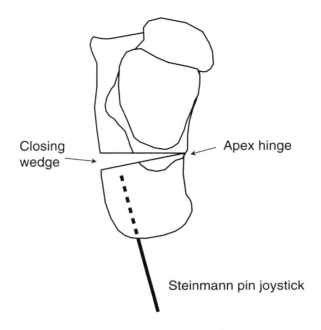

Closing wedge →

Apex hinge ←

Steinmann pin joystick

Completed closing wedge osteotomy

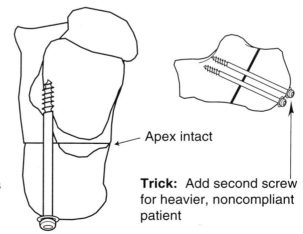

Apex intact ←

Only one 6.5 mm cancellous screw is needed because the apex is intact

Trick: Add second screw for heavier, noncompliant patient

Chapter 23
Gastrocnemius Slide

Stephen Pinney, M.D., M.Ed., F.R.C.S.(C.)
Sigvard T. Hansen Jr., M.D.

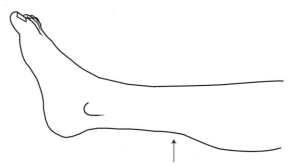

Flat area indicates junction of
gastrocnemius (gastroc) and soleus

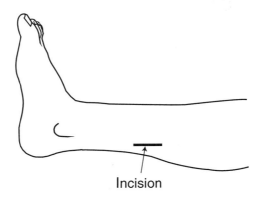

Incision

Identifying the Gastroc-soleus Interval

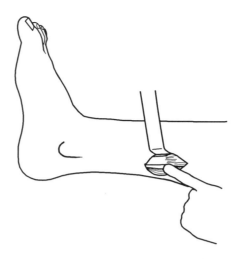

Developing the Gastroc-soleus Interval

Soleus fascia

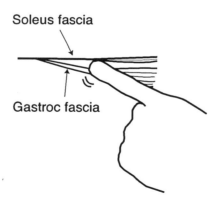

Gastroc fascia

Trick: Sweep finger proximally to find the gastroc muscle belly, then sweep down underneath it to find the gastroc-soleus interval

Identifying the Sural Nerve

Pitfall: Sural nerve may be stuck to gastroc fascia and cut during the release

Trick: Palpate the fascia for nerve. Gently separate above and below the release site

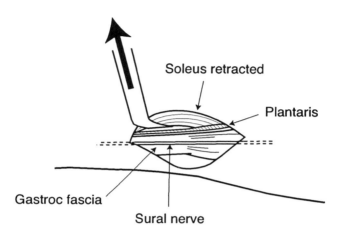

Soleus retracted

Plantaris

Gastroc fascia

Sural nerve

Dividing the Gastroc Fascia

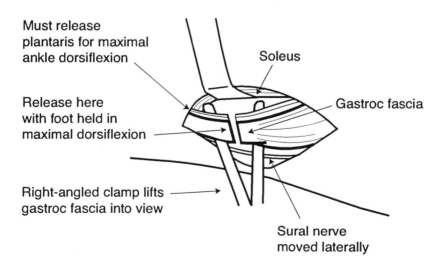

Must release plantaris for maximal ankle dorsiflexion

Release here with foot held in maximal dorsiflexion

Right-angled clamp lifts gastroc fascia into view

Soleus

Gastroc fascia

Sural nerve moved laterally

Checking the Adequacy of Release

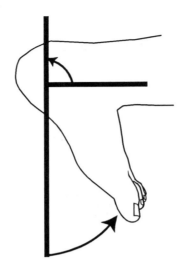

Ankle dorsiflexion is the
same regardless of
knee position

Stabilizing the Release

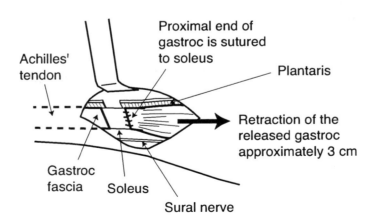

Proximal end of
gastroc is sutured
to soleus

Achilles'
tendon

Plantaris

Retraction of the
released gastroc
approximately 3 cm

Gastroc
fascia

Soleus

Sural nerve

Chapter 24 Adult Flatfoot Syndrome

Frederick G. Lippert III, M.D.
Sigvard T. Hansen Jr., M.D.

Features of Flat Foot Pathology

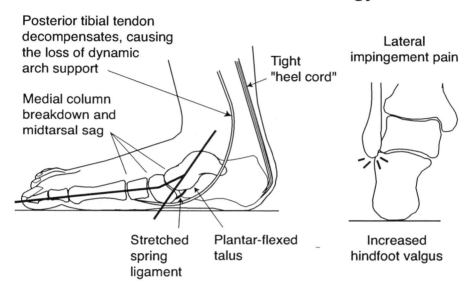

Posterior tibial tendon decompensates, causing the loss of dynamic arch support

Medial column breakdown and midtarsal sag

Tight "heel cord"

Lateral impingement pain

Stretched spring ligament

Plantar-flexed talus

Increased hindfoot valgus

Determining the Contribution of the Gastrocnemius and Soleus to a "Tight Heel Cord"

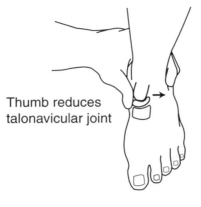

Thumb reduces talonavicular joint

Foot reduced and held during range of motion

Note: Acceptable dorsiflexion depends on the health of the foot/ankle tissues, presenting problem, and severity

Example: Healthy runner with no foot problems and no dorsiflexion does not require release

Example: Midfoot DJD requires 25^0 to 30^0 dorsiflexion from the release to protect the mid-foot

Tight gastrocnemius only

Tight gastrocnemius and soleus

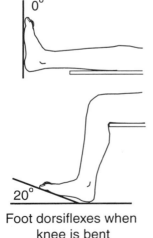

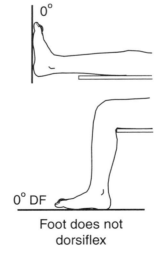

Foot dorsiflexes when knee is bent

Foot does not dorsiflex

Medial Column Changes Seen on a Weightbearing X-Ray

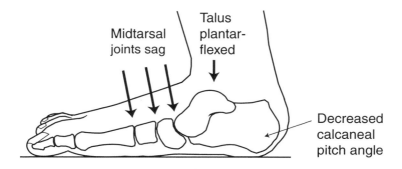

Midtarsal joints sag

Talus plantar-flexed

Decreased calcaneal pitch angle

Pitfall: Nonweightbearing lateral foot X-rays may look normal

Trick: Take weightbearing lateral X-rays with knee extended and 10° forward lean. Use axes as reference for assessing deformity

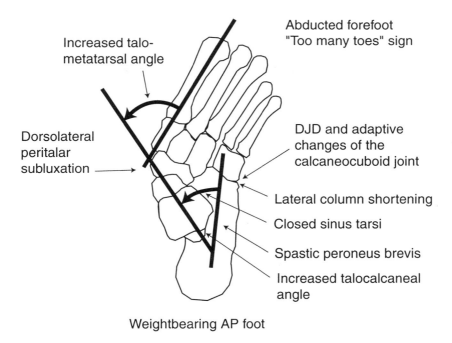

Increased talo-metatarsal angle

Abducted forefoot "Too many toes" sign

Dorsolateral peritalar subluxation

DJD and adaptive changes of the calcaneocuboid joint

Lateral column shortening

Closed sinus tarsi

Spastic peroneus brevis

Increased talocalcaneal angle

Weightbearing AP foot

Procedures for Stage II Flat Foot Surgery

Medial Calcaneal Osteotomy

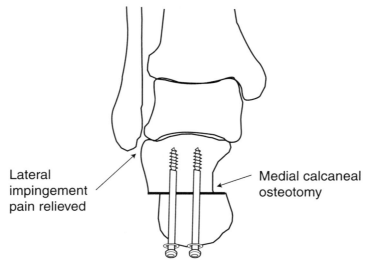

Lateral impingement pain relieved

Medial calcaneal osteotomy

Decreased hindfoot valgus

Check alignment in the operating room

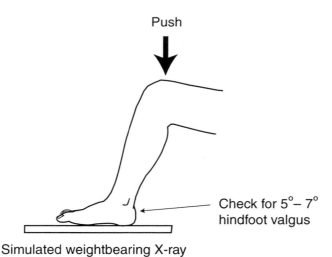

Push

Check for 5°– 7° hindfoot valgus

Simulated weightbearing X-ray

Medial Column Stabilization

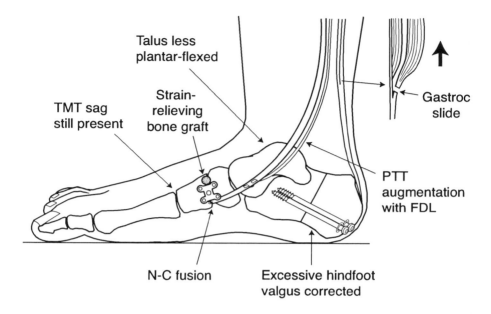

Talus less plantar-flexed

Strain-relieving bone graft

TMT sag still present

Gastroc slide

PTT augmentation with FDL

N-C fusion

Excessive hindfoot valgus corrected

Pitfall: Releasing the entire heel cord when only gastrocnemius is tight causes prolonged plantarflexion weakness

Trick: Evaluate gastroc-soleus individually for tightness using knee-flexion test. Release only gastroc fascia

Trick: Use at least two screws across each joint surface

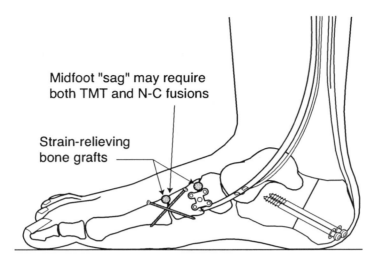

Midfoot "sag" may require both TMT and N-C fusions

Strain-relieving bone grafts

Trick: Do all required procedures at the same time rather than individually over time

Alternate Fixation for TMT and N-C Fusions

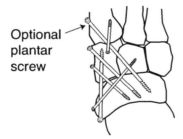

Optional plantar screw

Lateral Column Lengthening

Trick: Use at least two screws across each fusion surface

Pitfall: Screws alone break, so use with H plate, but plates may cause irritation of tendons and soft tissue

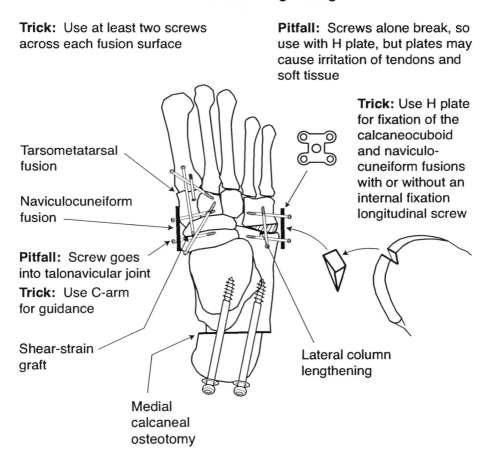

Trick: Use H plate for fixation of the calcaneocuboid and naviculo-cuneiform fusions with or without an internal fixation longitudinal screw

Tarsometatarsal fusion

Naviculocuneiform fusion

Pitfall: Screw goes into talonavicular joint

Trick: Use C-arm for guidance

Shear-strain graft

Lateral column lengthening

Medial calcaneal osteotomy

Pitfalls:
1. Overcorrection to cavovarus by maximally opening calcaneocuboid joint with lamina spreaders
2. Excessive stripping of N-C and C-C joints risks nonunion

Tricks:
1. Open only until T-N joint is congruent
2. Limit stripping. Add shear-strain graft

Procedure for Stage III Flat Foot Surgery
Triple Arthrodesis

Goal: Achieve at least 5° to 7° hindfoot valgus

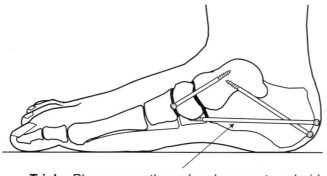

Pitfall: Poor calcaneocuboid screw purchase

Trick: Place screw through calcaneus to cuboid

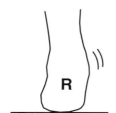

Pitfall: Dynamic hind foot roll out due to hindfoot varus

Trick: Tell patient preoperatively that a calcaneal osteotomy may be needed later to fine tune hindfoot alignment

Alternate technique for extending the fusion to midfoot

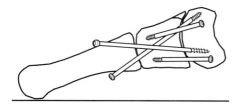 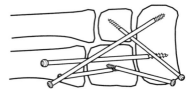

Chapter 25 Pes Cavus

Sigvard T. Hansen Jr., M.D.
Frederick G. Lippert III, M.D.

Calcaneus Deformity

Problem: EDL and EHL overpower weak gastroc-soleus. PT and PL work as ankle flexors

Solution: Transfer all functioning flexors to Achilles tendon

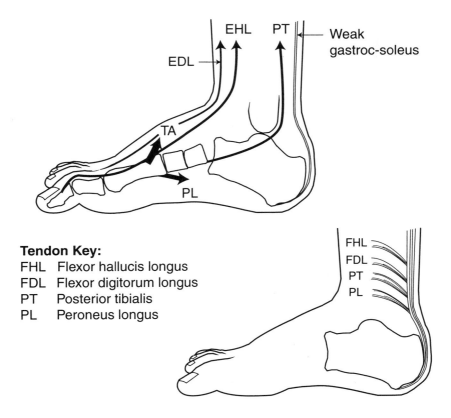

Tendon Key:
FHL Flexor hallucis longus
FDL Flexor digitorum longus
PT   Posterior tibialis
PL   Peroneus longus

Trick: Transfer tendons causing deformity first
Example: PL to Achilles tendon when 5 + strength and plantar-flexing first ray. PT to Achilles tendon when it is inverting the foot

The Coleman Block Test

The Coleman block test is used to distinguish hindfoot-driven cavus from forefoot-driven cavus. With hindfoot-driven cavus, the hindfoot is fixed and the forefoot is mobile. With forefoot-driven cavus, the forefoot is fixed and the hindfoot is mobile.

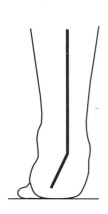 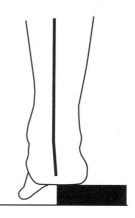 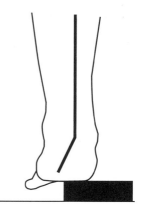

Right
hindfoot varus

Forefoot-driven varus
• Forefoot rigid
  hindfoot mobile
• Hindfoot varus
  moves to valgus

Hindfoot-driven varus
• Forefoot mobile
  hindfoot rigid
• Hindfoot remains
  in varus

Correcting Hindfoot-Driven Varus

Problem: Posterior tibialis overpowers PB. Fixed hindfoot cavovarus

Trick: Neutralize PT and lateralize hindfoot. PT transfered to the tibialis anterior or lateral foot depending on muscle imbalance

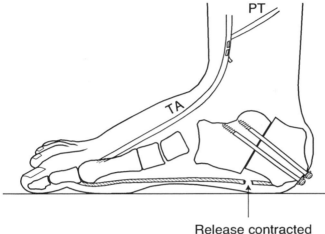

PT

TA

Pitfall: Forefoot varus if PT is attached too medial

Release contracted plantar fascia

Trick: Valgus calcaneal osteotomy to restore hindfoot alignment. Dorsal slide to decrease hindfoot cavus

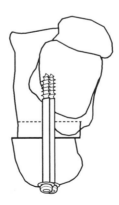

Correcting Forefoot-Driven Hindfoot Varus

Problem: PL overpowers TA causing plantar-flexed first metatarsal and claw toe

Pitfall: Patient may have both forefoot and hindfoot cavus (i.e., Charcot-Marie-Tooth Disease)

Trick: For rigid plantar-flexed first metatarsal, do a dorsal closing wedge osteotomy

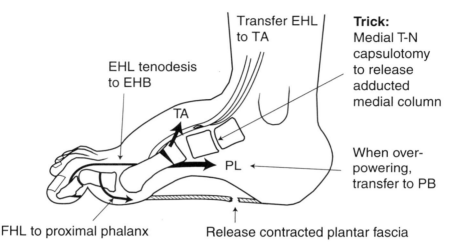

Trick: EHL and FHL tendon transfers to correct claw toe deformity

Trick: Transfer PL to PB

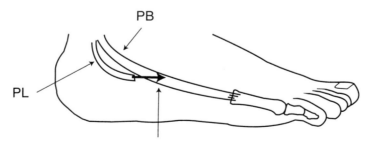

Trick: Release PL here and transfer to PB

Completed Correction of
Mixed Cavovarus Deformities

Trick: Compensatory deformation may require a mixture of forefoot and hindfoot procedures

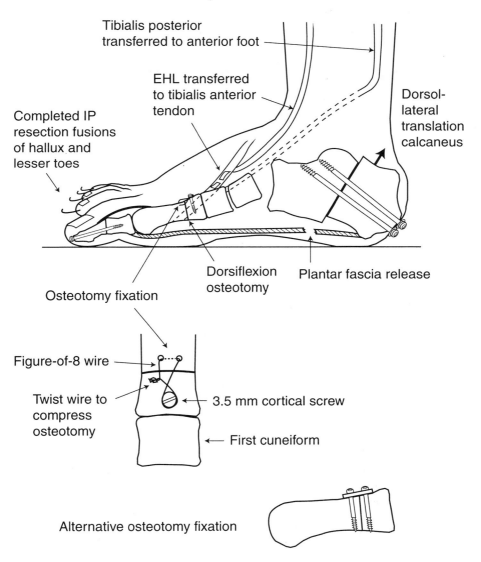

Tibialis posterior transferred to anterior foot

EHL transferred to tibialis anterior tendon

Completed IP resection fusions of hallux and lesser toes

Dorsolateral translation calcaneus

Osteotomy fixation

Dorsiflexion osteotomy

Plantar fascia release

Figure-of-8 wire

Twist wire to compress osteotomy

3.5 mm cortical screw

First cuneiform

Alternative osteotomy fixation

Chapter 26
Haglund's Deformity and Insertional Achilles Tendinosis

Frederick G. Lippert III, M.D.
Sigvard T. Hansen Jr., M.D.

Debridement of Haglund's Deformity and Insertional Tendinosis

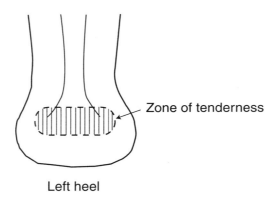

Zone of tenderness

Left heel

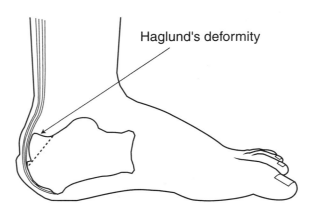

Haglund's deformity

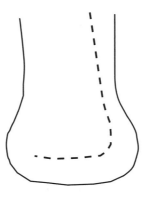

Skin incision

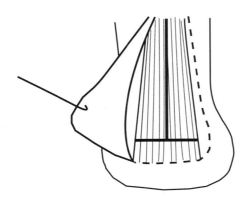

Tendon incision

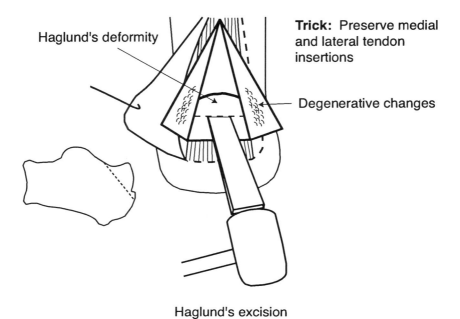

Haglund's deformity

Trick: Preserve medial and lateral tendon insertions

Degenerative changes

Haglund's excision

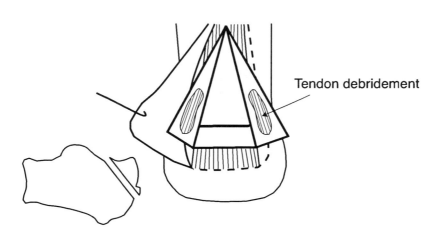

Tendon debridement

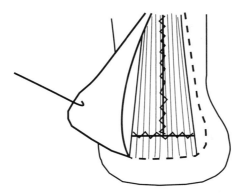

Tendon closure

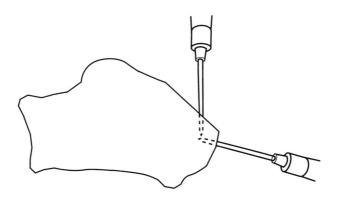

Technique for hole placement for sutures

Tendon closure

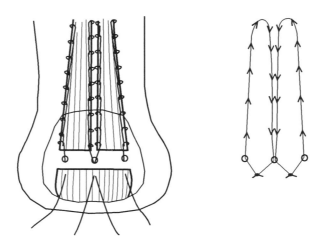

Tendon attachment to bone using Krackow stitch

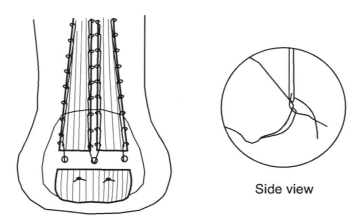

Side view

Chapter 27
Brostrom Procedure for
Chronic Ankle Laxity

Frederick G. Lippert III, M.D.
Sigvard T. Hansen Jr., M.D.

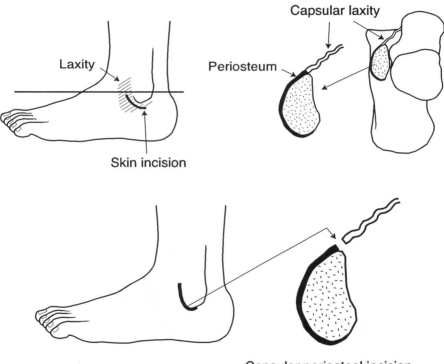

Transverse plane of the fibula at the ankle level

Capsular laxity

Laxity

Periosteum

Skin incision

Capsular periosteal incision

Pitfall: Capsule attenuated, repair will stretch out

Trick: Do a peroneus brevis, lesser toe extensor, or plantaris tendon weave reconstruction

Bone surface abraded to improve capsular attachment

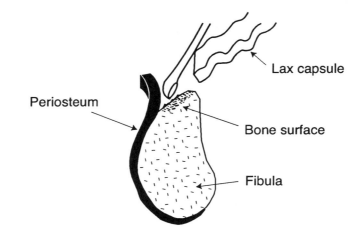

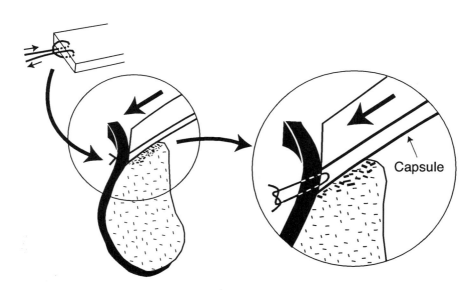

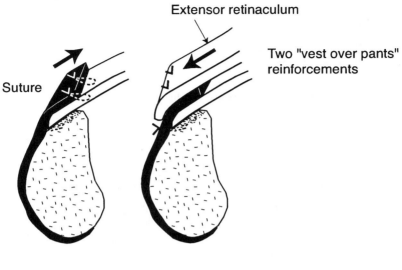

Suture

Extensor retinaculum

Two "vest over pants" reinforcements

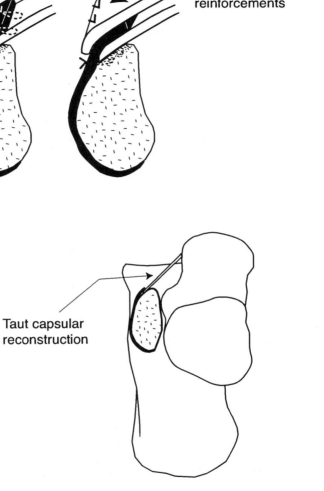

Taut capsular reconstruction

Chapter 28 Redo Brostrom for Failed Primary Brostrom and Other Ligament Surgery

Frederick G. Lippert III, M.D.
Sigvard T. Hansen Jr., M.D.

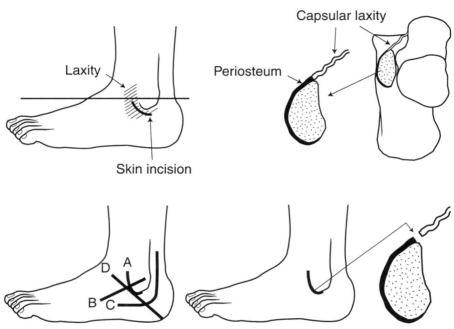

Transverse plane of the fibula at the ankle level

Original capsular periosteal incision

Index:
A. Incision okay to use again when redo is likely
B. Incision when combined with calcaneal osteotomy
C. Incision when Chrisman-Snook tendon weave is possible
D. Incision along skin lines—extensile exposure

Pitfall: Not addressing predisposing problems
1. Hindfoot varus
2. Tight gastrocnemius

Problem: Attenuated periosteal layer
Trick: Cover with capsular flap

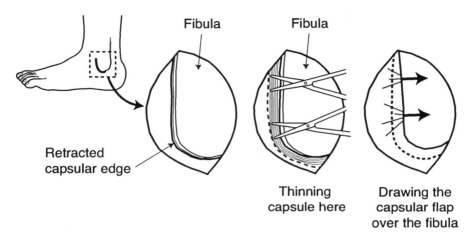

Fibula

Fibula

Retracted
capsular edge

Thinning
capsule here

Drawing the
capsular flap
over the fibula

Problem: Attenuated capsular flap
Trick: Reconstitute capsular flap. Create overlapping flaps to cover defect

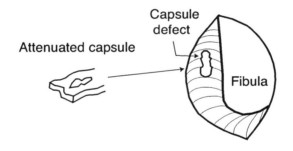

Capsule
defect

Attenuated capsule

Fibula

Capsular defect quartered

Quartered flaps interdigitated

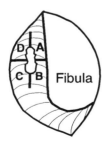

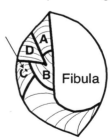

Chapter 28 Redo Brostrom for Failed
Primary Brostrom and Other Ligament Surgery   115

Anatomy of the Redo Brostrom

Pitfall: Abbreviated or missing tissue
Trick: Overlap with scar tissue and retinaculum

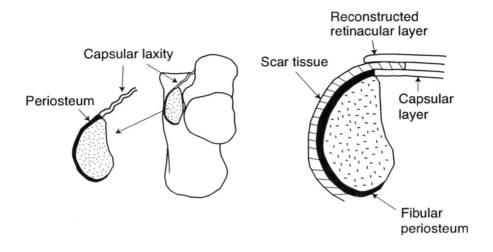

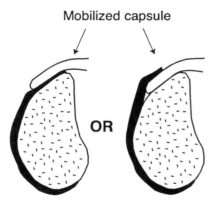

Trick: Mobilize capsular flap to articulate with available periosteum

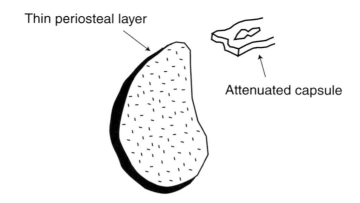

Thin periosteal layer

Attenuated capsule

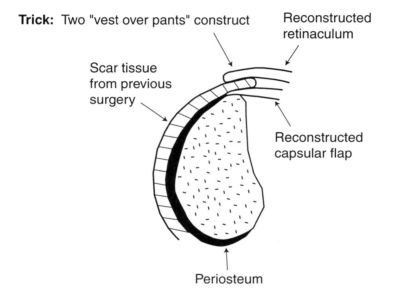

Trick: Two "vest over pants" construct

Reconstructed retinaculum

Scar tissue from previous surgery

Reconstructed capsular flap

Periosteum

Pitfalls:
1. Sutures pull through tissue
2. Flimsy construct

Trick: Abort redo and substitute tendon weave reconstruction

Chapter 29
Peroneal Tendon Subluxation

Frederick G. Lippert III, M.D.
Sigvard T. Hansen Jr., M.D.

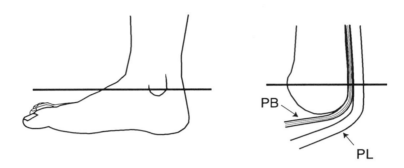

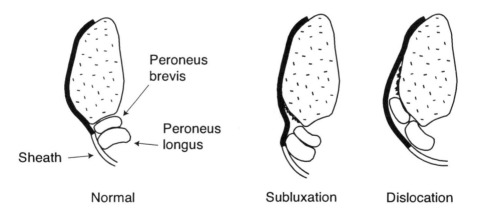

Retinacular separation from fibula

Peroneus brevis

Peroneus longus

Sheath

Normal

Subluxation

Dislocation

Treatment of Peroneal Tendon Subluxation

Retinacular Reconstruction
with Slip from Achilles or Plantaris Tendon

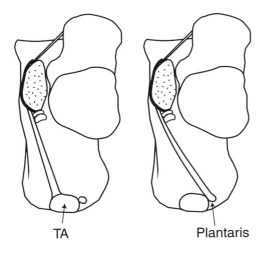

TA   Plantaris

Deepening tendon groove

Remove bone

Elevate cartilage

Pitfall: Restricted dorsiflexion due to short length of strip

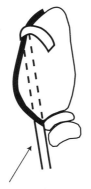

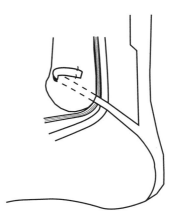

Tendon slip from Achilles' or plantaris prevents subluxation or dislocation

Trick: Harvest slightly more than needed

Chapter 30 Calcaneus Fractures and Fixation Techniques

Paul J. Juliano, M.D.

Fracture Pattern

Calcaneus fracture pattern lateral view

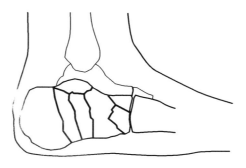

Typical calcaneal fracture pattern coronal view

Impacted posterior facet

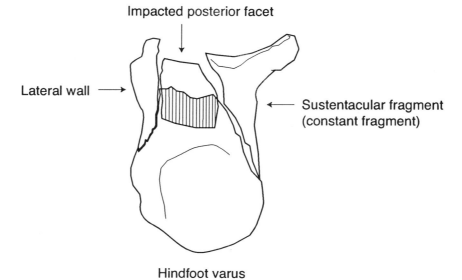

Lateral wall ⟶

⟵ Sustentacular fragment (constant fragment)

Hindfoot varus

Setup for monitoring fracture reduction and internal fixation

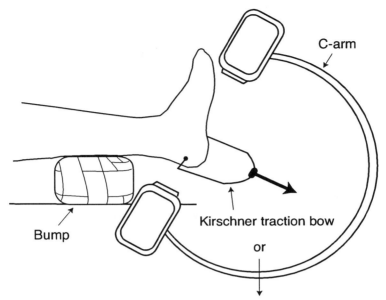

C-arm

Bump

Kirschner traction bow

or

Schantz pin on T-handle with comminution of tuberosity

Surgical exposure

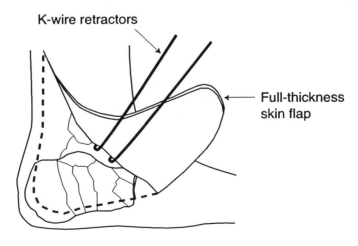

K-wire retractors

Full-thickness skin flap

Chapter 30 Calcaneus Fractures and Fixation Techniques   121

Fracture Reduction

Disimpacting the fracture

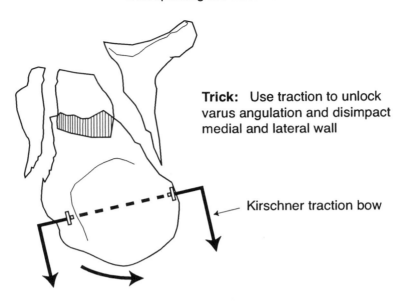

Trick: Use traction to unlock varus angulation and disimpact medial and lateral wall

Kirschner traction bow

Reduction of Posterior Facet

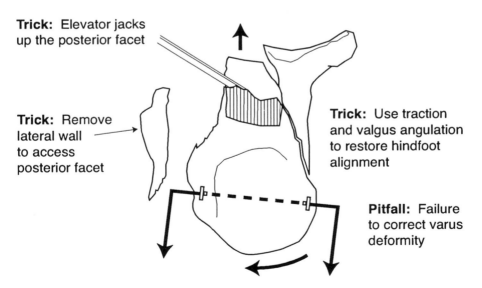

Trick: Elevator jacks up the posterior facet

Trick: Remove lateral wall to access posterior facet

Trick: Use traction and valgus angulation to restore hindfoot alignment

Pitfall: Failure to correct varus deformity

Fracture Reduced

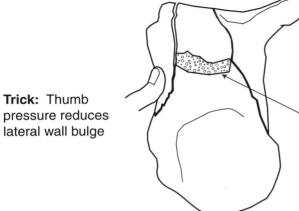

Trick: Thumb pressure reduces lateral wall bulge

Pitfall: Residual defect is left when the impacted posterior facet is elevated to anatomic position

Provisional Fixation

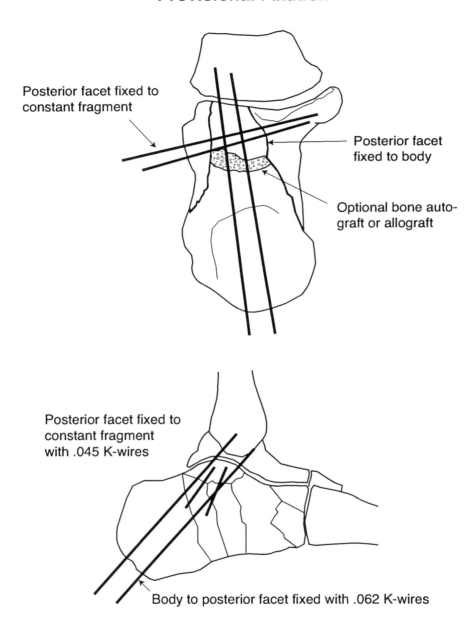

Posterior facet fixed to constant fragment

Posterior facet fixed to body

Optional bone auto-graft or allograft

Posterior facet fixed to constant fragment with .045 K-wires

Body to posterior facet fixed with .062 K-wires

Completed Fixation

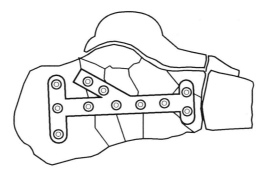

Calcaneal fracture fixed with calcaneal plate and screws

Trick: Fully threaded smaller cortical screws provide better bite (2.7 – 3.5 mm). Must lag with glide hole

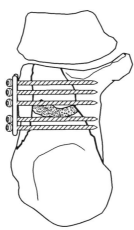

Pitfalls:

40 cancellous lag screws
1. Difficult removal due to no back cutting
2. Large threads don't grip small fragments
3. Screw failure when junction near fracture line (shear line)

Cannulated screws
1. Expensive
2. Guide-system problems
3. Large screw heads
4. Reduced bite

Hardware Placement for Primary Subtalar Fusion

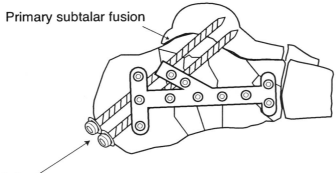

Primary subtalar fusion

Trick:
1. Use fully threaded screws to prevent collapse
2. May use one 6.5 mm and one 3.5 mm screw for smaller area

Chapter 31 Percutaneous Pinning of Talar Neck Fractures

Paul J. Juliano, M.D.
Amir Fayazi, M.D.

Step 1: Insert Traction Pin in the Calcaneus

1. Talus subluxed posteriorly on calcaneus

2. Calcaneus pin inserted

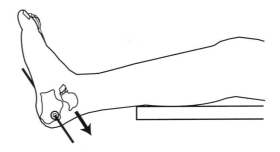

Step 2: Manipulation for Type III Hawkins Fracture

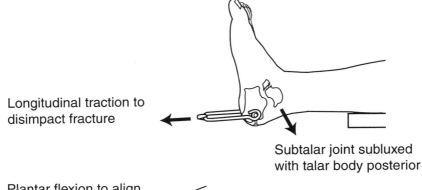

Longitudinal traction to disimpact fracture

Subtalar joint subluxed with talar body posterior

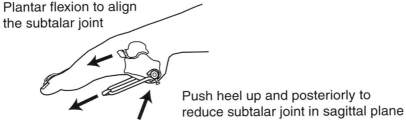

Plantar flexion to align the subtalar joint

Push heel up and posteriorly to reduce subtalar joint in sagittal plane

Dorsiflex Foot to Neutral

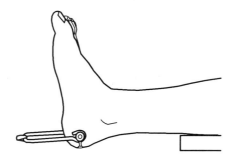

Medial 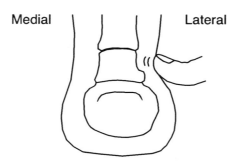 Lateral

Thumb pressure used to fine tune
subtalar reduction in coronal plane

Canale view X-ray

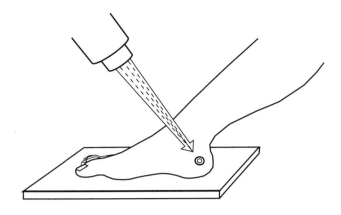

Pins are placed using a biplanar fluoroscope

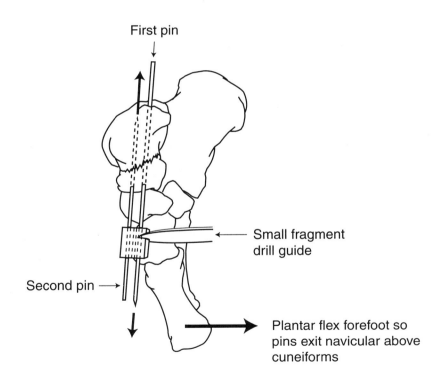

First pin

Small fragment
drill guide

Second pin →

Plantar flex forefoot so
pins exit navicular above
cuneiforms

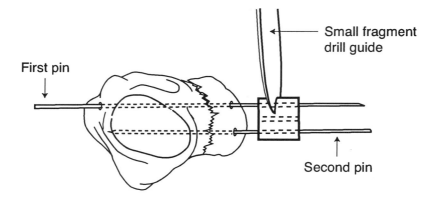

First pin

Small fragment
drill guide

Second pin

Okay for second screw threads to cross fracture since the first screw
has compressed the fracture

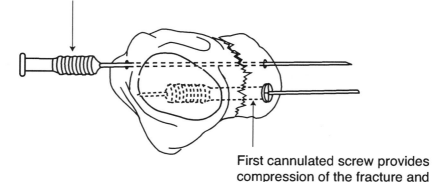

First cannulated screw provides
compression of the fracture and
must be countersunk

Chapter 32 LisFranc Dislocation

Edward S. Holt, M.D.

Percutaneous Internal Fixation Using 3.5 mm Cannulated Screws

Key Points:

1. TMT flexion injuries – dorsal ligament disruption only – temporary screw technique; screws removed after 12 weeks
2. Usually fix TMT joints 1 through 3 but may fix only TMT 1 and 2 with intact plantar ligaments
3. For TMT-displaced injuries with disruption of plantar ligaments use primary fusion

Trick: Place this guide wire dorsal to the first one

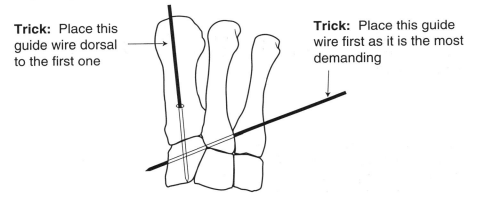

Trick: Place this guide wire first as it is the most demanding

Pitfall: Loss of anatomic reduction of the second TMT during guide wire placement prevents a good result. Don't think "the screw will pull it together." Observe alignment with a C-arm

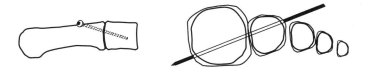

Trick: Aim this guide wire 20° to 30° plantar to hold the second metatarsal down

Trick: Gastrocnemius slide to protect plantar ligaments

Percutaneous Screw Removal

Trick: Select the second metatarsal screw such that it protrudes 8 to 10 mm beyond the medial cuneiform. Also punch the guide wire through the skin to create a small scar. This will enable you to relocate this screw for removal later

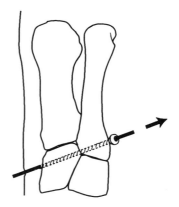

Pitfall: If the screw is too long and it tents the skin tightly, it may erode through before removal. If it is too short, you can't feel it later. It should be easily palpated

Trick: When removing the screw, anesthetize the skin over the tip of the screw with a very small amount of local, then puncture the skin with a sterile guide wire and pass the wire retrograde through the screw until it can be located through the old dorsal incision. Remove the screw with a cannulated screwdriver over the wire. The first TMT screw is easily located and removed with a guide wire and cannulated screwdriver in the usual fashion

Pitfall: Too much local anesthesia over the tip of the screw can make it quite difficult to locate

Chapter 33 Subtalar Arthrodesis

Frederick G. Lippert III, M.D.
Sigvard T. Hansen Jr., M.D.

Trick: Preparation of surfaces

Remove only cartilage. Preserve subchondral bone and joint surfaces for best coaptation of surfaces. Rotate talus on calcaneus to achieve 7° hindfoot valgus

1. Use straight and curved osteotomes to pry open the subtalar joint, mobilize the talus, and remove all cartilage down to the subchondral bone

2. Use straight and down-biting curettes to remove remote surfaces such as the back of the posterior facet

3. Drill subchondral bone to connect the marrow cavity with the fusion site

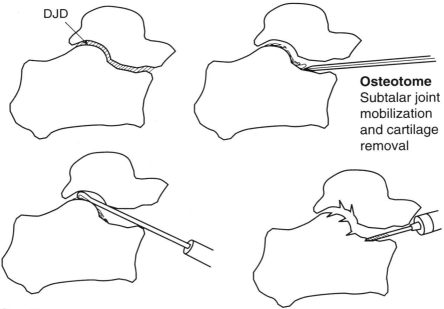

DJD

Osteotome
Subtalar joint mobilization and cartilage removal

Curette
1. Cartilage removed from posterior facet
2. Subchondral bone preserved

Drill
Subchondral bone penetrated to promote fusion

Correction of Hindfoot Alignment

Concept: Mobilize subtalar joint and rotate the talus on the calcaneus to obtain the desired amount of hindfoot valgus – lateral rotation to decrease hindfoot valgus and internal rotation to increase hindfoot valgus

Pitfall: Failure to adequately mobilize subtalar joint results in incomplete correction of hindfoot alignment

Trick: Correct deformity and achieve desired hindfoot position by moving the talus on the calcaneus. Avoid taking wedges, which shortens the foot

Trick: Check hindfoot alignment
1. Raise leg and look up back of ankle
2. Use simulated weightbearing X-ray to look at talocalcaneal and talometatarsal angle
3. Feel how foot sits on X-ray plate
4. Put tip of index finger in center of heel pad and note alignment with long axis of tibia, lateral to axis hindfoot valgus, medial to axis hindfoot varus

Trick: Mobilize subtalar joint
1. Open sustentacular capsule and remove medial facet cartilage
2. Smooth lateral articular margins of posterior facet joint
3. Push hindfoot with thumb

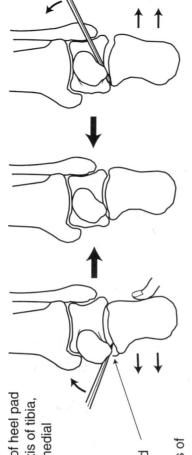

Valgus deformity   Normal   Varus deformity

Fixation

Temporary pin fixation

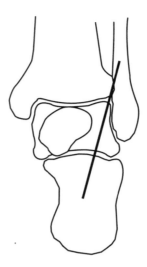

Permanent Screw Fixation

Trick: Place foot on C-arm in lateral position for screw guidance

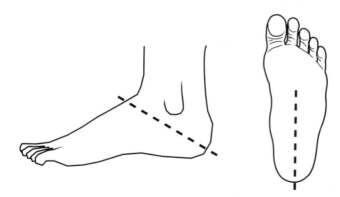

Trick: Place screws by reference to skin markings

Skin markings represent desired screw placement in two planes. Surgeon drills screw holes using these lines as a reference

Alternative Methods to Guide Drill Direction

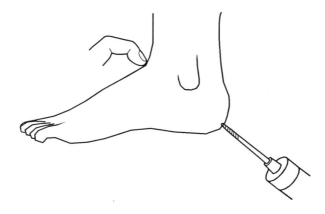

Trick: Place screws by reference to anatomic landmarks.
Surgeon guides drill by aiming for the tip of an index finger placed
over the base of the neck of the talus

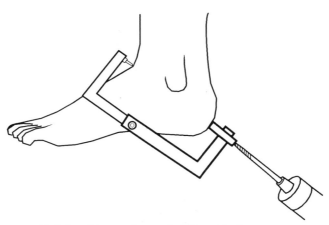

Trick: Use universal drill guide for
screw placement

Sequence of Screw Placement

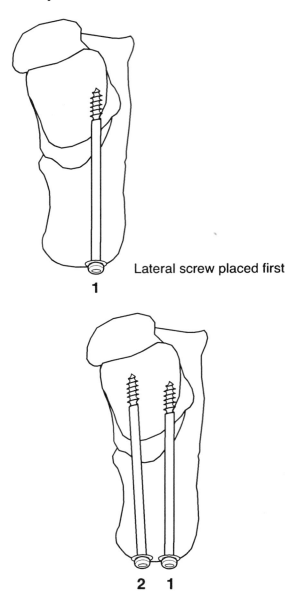

Lateral screw placed first

1

Medial screw into talar neck placed second using first screw as reference

Ideal Screw Placement

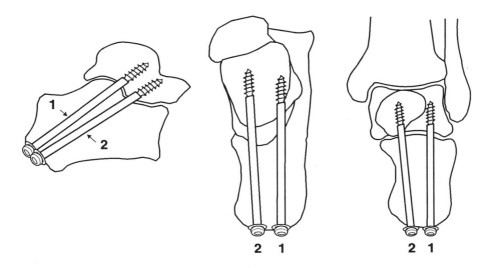

Pitfall: Single screw close to the axis of rotation results in no rotational control

Trick: Use two screws across subtalar joint

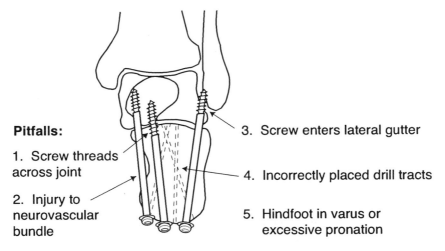

Pitfalls:

1. Screw threads across joint

2. Injury to neurovascular bundle

3. Screw enters lateral gutter

4. Incorrectly placed drill tracts

5. Hindfoot in varus or excessive pronation

Trick: "Push" the screw medially when drilling lateral screw hole

Chapter 34 Subtalar Arthrodesis with Alternate Screw Placement

Edward S. Holt, M.D.

Internal Fixation

Trick: Place screws in the best bone for screw purchase

Trick: First screw should be placed fairly medial in the calcaneus and talus

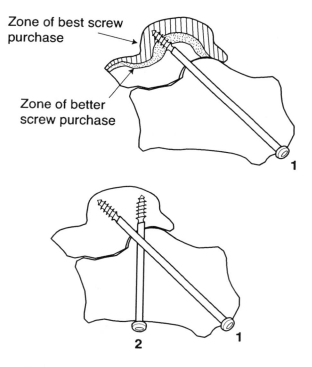

Trick: Place the second screw through the plantar lateral calcaneus just anterior to the heel pad. This can be done percutaneously with 6.5 or 7.3 mm cannulated screws. This fixation is remarkably sturdy and makes nonunion rare

Subtalar Fusion

Internal fixation

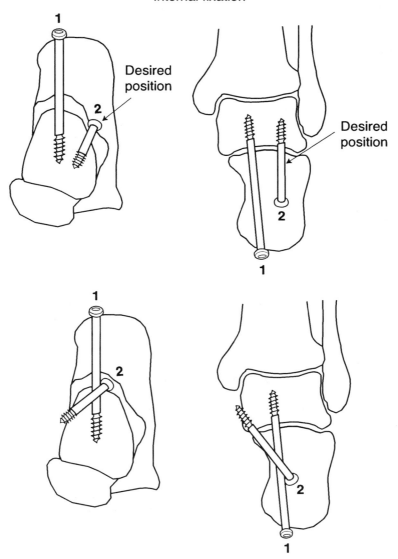

Pitfall: Make sure the second screw stays lateral to the first, otherwise it will tend to penetrate the medial talar wall. Use caution!

Index

Forefoot-driven hindfoot varus, correction protocols, 104